Cookbook for Beginners with Low Cholesterol

Amazing Plant-Based Recipes that are Delicious and Life-Changing

Traci R. Denton

Contents

Chapter One

BURGERS WITH BLACK BEANS AND VEGGIES MADE AT HOME

Approximately 35 minutes total time: 15 minutes for preparation, 20 minutes for cooking. Nutrient Facts: 198 calories | 33.1 grams of carbohydrates | 3 grams of fat | 11.2 grams of protein | 46 milligrams of cholesterol

INGREDIENTS

1. a 16-ounce can (drained and rinsed) of black beans

Chili powder (about 1 tablespoon)

1/4 of a green bell pepper, sliced into 2-inch chunks

14 cup cumin (or more)

onion, sliced into wedges (about half an onion)

1 teaspoon Thai chili sauce (or any spicy sauce of your choosing)

peeled and minced 3 garlic cloves

Breadcrumbs (about 1/2 cup).

Egg (a single one).

DIRECTIONS

Alternatively, prepare an outdoor grill to high heat and generously oil a layer of aluminum foil if cooking outside. Prepare the oven to 375 degrees F (190 degrees C) and gently oil a baking sheet if you choose to bake the desserts.

Mash black beans with a fork until they are thick and pasty in a medium-sized mixing dish.

Prepare the vegetables in a food processor by chopping them coarsely. Add this to the mashed beans and combine well.

Using a small mixing bowl, whisk together the egg, chili powder, cumin, and chili sauce until well combined.

Combine the crushed beans with the egg mixture. The mixture should be sticky and hold together after the bread crumbs have been added. Four patties should be formed from the ingredients.

Place patties on a baking sheet lined with aluminum foil and cook for approximately 8 minutes each side, if grilling. Place the patties on a baking sheet and bake for approximately 10 minutes on each side if you're going to bake them.

POTATOES THAT HAVE BEEN OVEN ROASTED.

Approximately 45 minutes total time: 15 minutes for preparation, 30 minutes for cooking. FACTS ABOUT VEGETABLE NUTRITION

289 calories | 53.1 grams of carbohydrate | 7.1 grams of fat | 5 grams of protein | 0 milligrams of cholesterol

INGREDIENTS

olive oil (eighth cup)

BURGERS WITH BLACK BEANS AND VEGGIES MADE AT HOME

oregano leaves (about 1/2 teaspoon)

1 tablespoon minced garlic, preferably fresh.

1/2 teaspoon dried parsley 1/2 teaspoon dry basil 1/2 teaspoon dried oregano 1/2 teaspoon dried oregano

a half teaspoon of red pepper flakes, finely chopped

1 teaspoon dried marjoram (optional).

a half teaspoon of salt and a half teaspoon of dill weed dried

Peeled and diced potatoes (four big potatoes)

1/2 teaspoon thyme leaves, dried

DIRECTIONS

400 degrees Fahrenheit for the oven (245 degrees C).

In a large mixing bowl, whisk together the oil, garlic, basil, marjoram, dill weed, thyme, oregano, parsley, red pepper flakes, and salt until well combined and well-flavored. Using a spatula, coat the potatoes evenly. Using a roasting pan or baking sheet, arrange the potatoes in a single layer.

Turning periodically, roast for 20 to 30 minutes in the preheated oven, until browned on both sides, depending on the size of the chicken.

PRETZEL TURTLES ARE A SPECIES OF TURTLES originating in the Pretzel region of Germany.

Preparation time: 10 minutes | Cooking time: 4 minutes | Total time: 14 minutes Servings: 20 FACTS ABOUT VEGETABLE NUTRITION

82 calories | 14.1 grams of carbohydrate | 2.2 grams of fat | 1.7 grams of protein | 1 milligrams of cholesterol

INGREDIENTS

tiny pretzels (about 20)

twenty half-shelled pecans

20 caramel candies dipped in chocolate

DIRECTIONS

Oven should be preheated to 300 degrees Fahrenheit (150 degrees C).

Prepare a cookie sheet with parchment paper and arrange the pretzels in a single layer on top of it. On each pretzel, place one caramel candy wrapped in chocolate.

4 minutes in the oven should enough. Whilst the candy is still warm, place a half-pecan onto each pretzel that has been coated with candy. Before keeping in an airtight container, allow the mixture to cool fully before handling.

RESTAURANT STYLE FRIED RICE CUISINE

Approximately 45 minutes total time: 15 minutes for preparation, 30 minutes for cooking, and 15 minutes for cleaning FACTS ABOUT VEGETABLE NUTRITION

261 calories | 39.7 grams of carbohydrate | 8.4 grams of fat | 5.8 grams of protein | 46 milligrams of cholesterol

INGREDIENTS

white rice, 2 cups (enriched)

Water in a 4-cup measuring cup 2 teaspoons vegetable oil egg whites (a total of 2)

Baby carrots (about a third of a cup) sliced

taste with a dash of soy sauce

BURGERS WITH BLACK BEANS AND VEGGIES MADE AT HOME

Sesame oil (to taste) 1/2 cup frozen green peas (optional)

DIRECTIONS

Rice and water are combined in a pot. To bring to a boil, put the water in a saucepan. Cover and simmer for 20 minutes on a low heat setting until vegetables are tender.

Cook carrots in water for 3 to 5 minutes in a small saucepan over medium heat. Drain the peas after they have been dropped into boiling water.

Using a high heat, warm the wok. Pour in the oil and toss in the carrots and peas for approximately 30 seconds, until the carrots are tender. To scramble the eggs with the veggies, crack them into the pan and stir briskly. Cooked rice should be added at this point. In a large mixing bowl, combine the soy sauce and rice and toss well. Toss the salad once more with sesame oil.

CURRY OF RED LENTILS

| Prep time: 10 minutes | Cooking time: 30 minutes | Total time: 40 minutes | 8 servings FACTS ABOUT VEGETABLE NUTRITION

Amount per serving: 192 calories, 32.5 grams of carbohydrates, 2.6 grams of fat, 12.1 grams of protein, and zero milligrams of cholesterol

INGREDIENTS

Red lentils (two cups)

Chili powder (around a teaspoon)

1 tablespoon vegetable oil 1 big onion (diced) 1 teaspoon salt

sugar (white) - 1 teaspoon

Curry Paste (about 2 tbsp.

1 teaspoon minced garlic, preferably fresh.

1 tbsp curry powder, to taste

Fresh ginger, finely chopped, 1 teaspoon

Turmeric powder (1 teaspoon)

a can of tomato puree (14.2 ounces)

1 teaspoon cumin seeds (ground)

DIRECTIONS

Using cold water, thoroughly rinse the lentils until the water runs clear. Using a large saucepan, fill the lentils with water to cover them and bring to a boil. Reduce heat to medium-low and simmer, adding more water as required to keep the lentils covered, for 15 to 20 minutes, or until the lentils are soft. Drain.

Cook and toss the onions in the heated oil for approximately 20 minutes, or until they are caramelized, in a large pan set over medium heat.

In a large mixing bowl, whisk together the curry paste, curry powder, turmeric, cumin, chili powder, salt, sugar, garlic, and ginger until well combined. Stir the mixture into the onions until well combined. Heat to high and cook, stirring regularly, for 1 to 2 minutes, or until the mixture smells pleasantly scented.

Remove the pan from the heat and mix in the tomato puree until it is fully incorporated.

BURRITO FILLING WITH SALSA CHICKEN

BURGERS WITH BLACK BEANS AND VEGGIES MADE AT HOME

Prepare: 5 minutes; cook: 30 minutes; total preparation and cooking time: 35 minutes. Nutrient Facts: 107 calories | 9.6 grams of carbohydrates | 1.5 grams of fat | 12.3 grams of protein • Cholesterol is 30 milligrams.

INGREDIENTS

chicken breast halves that have been skinned and boned

1 teaspoon cumin seeds (ground)

Tomato sauce (four-ounce can)

garlic, minced (about 2 cloves total)

salsa (a quarter cup)

Chili powder (around a teaspoon)

packet taco seasoning (about 1.25 ounces) sauce to taste in a small mixing bowl

DIRECTIONS

Over medium high heat, combine the chicken breasts and tomato sauce in a medium saucepan. Bring the water to a boil, then add the salsa, seasoning, cumin, garlic, and chili powder, and cook until the salsa is hot. Allow for a 15-minute simmering time period.

Pull the chicken flesh apart into thin threads using a fork, starting at one end. Using a lid, continue to simmer the pulled chicken flesh and sauce for another 5 to 10 minutes. In a large mixing bowl, combine all of the ingredients until well combined (Note: You may need to add a bit of water if the mixture is cooked too high and gets too thick.)

NOODLES OF ORZO AND GARLIC CHICKEN

Approximately 30 minutes total time: 15 minutes for preparation, 15 minutes for cooking. Nutritional Information: 351 calories; 40.4 grams of carbohydrates; 10.6 grams of fat; 22.3 grams of protein; 38 milligrams of cholesterol

INGREDIENTS

salt and pepper to taste, 1 cup uncooked orzo pasta, 2 tablespoons extra virgin olive oil

Fresh chopped parsley (about 1 teaspoon)

a garlic clove or two

Fresh spinach leaves (about 2)

crushed red pepper flakes (or grated) 1/4 teaspoon Topping with parmesan cheese

cut 2 skinless, boneless chicken breast halves into bite-size pieces each

DIRECTIONS

Start by filling a big saucepan halfway with lightly salted water and bringing it to a boil. Cook the orzo pasta for 8 to 10 minutes, or until it is al dente, before draining the water from the pot.

Cook the garlic and red pepper for 1 minute, or until the garlic turns golden brown, in a pan over medium-high heat until the oil is hot. Cook for 2 to 5 minutes, or until the chicken is lightly browned and the juices flow clear, stirring occasionally, until the chicken is done. Heat on medium-low for a few minutes, then add in the parsley and the orzo that has been cooked. Cooking the spinach in a pan is a great way to use up leftovers.

Allow the spinach to wilt for another 5 minutes while stirring periodically. To finish, sprinkle Parmesan cheese over top and serve immediately.

French Fries with Seasonings from Scratch (Homemade Crispy Seasoned Fries)

Preparation time: 15 minutes | Cooking time: 10 minutes | Total time: 25 minutes | 8 servings FACTS ABOUT VEGETABLE NUTRITION

Amount per serving: 192 calories | 378 grams of carbohydrates | 3.1 grams of fat | 3.9 grams of protein | zero milligrams of cholesterol

INGREDIENTS

peeling and dicing two and a half pounds russet potatoes

salt, 1 cup all-purpose flour, and a few more ingredients

1-tsp. paprika, to taste

garlic salt (around 1 tsp.

as required, up to 1/2 cup water

salt (onion) to taste, 1 teaspoon

cooking oil (vegetable or canola) 1 cup

DIRECTIONS

In a large mixing bowl, combine the potatoes, salt, and pepper. Stir until the potatoes are evenly coated with the salt and pepper.

Over medium-high heat, warm the oil in a large skillet. Meanwhile, sprinkle the flour, garlic salt, onion salt, normal salt, and paprika into a large mixing basin while the oil is heated. Stir in just enough water to make the mixture thin enough to trickle from a spoon, one teaspoon at a time.

Potato slices should be dipped into the batter one at a time and placed in the heated oil so that they do not contact each other at the start of the cooking process. To prevent the fries from clumping together, they must be put into the pan one at a time. Fry until golden brown and crispy, about 3 minutes each batch. To remove, use paper towels to soak up the excess moisture.

MEATLOAF CUPS WITH TURKEY AND VEGGIE

Prepare for ten servings in twenty minutes, cook for twenty-five minutes, and total fifty minutes. FACTS ABOUT VEGETABLE NUTRITION

119 calories | 13.6 grams of carbohydrate | 1 gram of fat | 13.2 grams of protein | 47 milligrams of cholesterol

INGREDIENTS

3 eggs, 1 1/2 cups coarsely chopped onions, 2 cups finely sliced zucchini

2-tbl. Worcestershire sauce (optional)

finely sliced 1 small red bell pepper

1 tbsp. Dijon mustard, grated

Extra-lean ground turkey (about 1 pound)

or as much as you need of the barbecue sauce

uncooked Couscous (half a cup uncooked)

DIRECTIONS

BURGERS WITH BLACK BEANS AND VEGGIES MADE AT HOME

Bake at 400 degrees Fahrenheit for 20 minutes (200 degrees C). Cooking spray should be sprayed into 20 muffin tins.

Using a food processor, pulse several times until the zucchini, onions, and red bell pepper are finely diced but not liquefied, about 30 seconds. In a large mixing bowl, combine the veggies with the ground turkey, couscous, egg, Worcestershire sauce, and Dijon mustard until everything is well mixed. About 3/4 of the way fill each prepared muffin cup. Approximately 1 teaspoon barbecue sauce should be placed on top of each cup.

25 minutes or until the juices flow clear in the preheated oven, depending on the size of your bird. Instant-read meat thermometer readings of the inside of a muffin should be at least 160 degrees Fahrenheit (70 degrees Celsius) (70 degrees C). Allow for a 5-minute resting period before preparing to serve.

CARROTS WITH PAT'S COOKED BEANS

1 hour and 30 minutes total time for 10 servings (preparation, cooking and cleanup). FACTS ABOUT VEGETABLE NUTRITION

399 calories | 68 grams of carbohydrate | 9.1 grams of fat | 14.1 grams of protein | 12 milligrams of cholesterol

INGREDIENTS

7 strips bacon, cut into 6 slices

Drain and rinse one (15-ounce) can garbanzo beans.

chopped onion (about one cup)

Ketchup (a quarter of a cup)

1 minced garlic clove (about 1 clove total)

Molasses (1/2 cup)

Can of pinto beans, 16 ounces

4 tablespoons of brown sugar that has been sealed

Great Northern beans, one (16-ounce) can (with the liquid removed)

2-tbl. Worcestershire sauce (optional)

1. Baked beans, one (16-ounce) can

1/4 cup dry mustard (yellow)

half a teaspoon ground pepper 1 (16-ounce) can red kidney beans, drained

DIRECTIONS

Oven should be preheated to 375 degrees Fahrenheit (190 degrees C).

A large, deep skillet is ideal for cooking bacon. Continue to cook until evenly browned over medium-high heat. Set aside in a large mixing bowl after draining and reserving 2 tablespoons of drippings. Cook the onion and garlic in the reserved bacon drippings until the onion is tender, then drain excess grease and transfer to a large mixing bowl with the bacon and parsley to combine.

Pinto beans, northern beans, baked beans, kidney beans, and garbanzo beans can be added to the bacon and onions. Combine the ketchup, molasses, brown sugar, Worcestershire sauce, mustard, and black pepper in a large mixing bowl until well combined. In a 9x12 inch casserole dish, combine all of the ingredients until well combined.

Wrap tightly in aluminum foil and bake for 1 hour in a preheated oven.

BLACK BEANS WITHOUT A DOUBT

Approximately 15 minutes total: 10 minutes for preparation, 5 minutes for cooking. FACTS ABOUT VEGETABLE NUTRITION

Amount per serving: 112 calories, 20.8 grams of carbohydrates, 0.4 grams of fat, 7 grams of protein, and zero milligrams of cholesterol

INGREDIENTS

Black beans (1 can, 16 ounces)

cilantro, chopped (about a tablespoon)

1/4 teaspoon cayenne pepper 1 small onion, finely diced

chopped 1 large onion, salt to taste 1 clove garlic, minced

Cook the beans, onion, and garlic in a medium saucepan until the beans are tender but not overcooked. Reduce the heat to medium-low and continue to cook until done. cilantro, cayenne pepper, and salt are all optional seasonings. Remove from heat and set aside for 5 minutes before serving.

BAKING ZUCCHINI CHIPS IN A SHORT AMOUNT OF TIME.

Prepare for four servings in five minutes. Cook for ten minutes. Nutritional Information: 92 calories; 13.8 grams of carbohydrate; 1.7 grams of fat; 6.1 grams of protein; and 2 milligrams of cholesterol

INGREDIENTS

2 medium zucchini, thinly sliced (about 1/4 inch thick).

2 tbsp. grated Parmesan cheese (optional).

1/2 cup dry bread crumbs that have been seasoned.

the whites of 2 eggs

peppercorns, ground to a fine powder

DIRECTIONS

475 degrees Fahrenheit should be set for the oven (245 degrees C).

Then, combine the bread crumbs with the pepper and Parmesan cheese in a small bowl. Using a separate bowl, whisk together the egg whites. Breadcrumbs are coated with egg whites and then dipped into breadcrumb mixture. Lay out on a baking sheet that has been greased.

After 5 minutes in the preheated oven, flip the pan and bake for another 5 to 10 minutes, until the bottom is browned and crisp.

SPICY BLACK-EYED PEAS COOKED ON THE LOW SETTING

| Prep time: 30 minutes | Cooking time: 6 hours and 30 minutes | Total time: 6 hours and 30 minutes | FACTS ABOUT VEGETABLE NUTRITION

Amount per serving: 199 calories, 30.2 grams of carbohydrate, 2.9 grams of fat, 14.1 grams of protein, 10 milligrams of cholesterol

INGREDIENTS

water, 8 ounces diced ham, 6 cups

1 cube chicken bouillon cube (optional).

BURGERS WITH BLACK BEANS AND VEGGIES MADE AT HOME

bacon, chopped (four slices)

I used 1 pound dried black-eyed peas, which I separated and rinsed.

a half teaspoon of cayenne pepper (optional)

onion, diced (about 1 onion)

1/4 cup cumin (approximately).

1 red bell pepper, stemmed, seeded, and diced 2 cloves garlic, diced salt to taste 1 red onion, minced

black pepper (ground) 1 teaspoon

seeds and minced 1 jalapeno chile (optional)

INSTRUCTIONS 1. Fill a slow cooker halfway with water and add the bouillon cube, stirring to dissolve. In a large mixing bowl, combine the black-eyed peas with the onion, garlic, bell pepper with jalapeno pepper, ham and bacon with the cayenne pepper, cumin, salt, and pepper; stir well. Cook on Low for 6 to 8 hours, or until the beans are tender, covered in the slow cooker on the stovetop.

RICE AND CARROT

| Preparation time: 15 minutes | Cooking time: 20 minutes | Total preparation time: 35 minutes. FACTS ABOUT VEGETABLE NUTRITION

Nutritious and low in cholesterol, this dish has only 179 calories, 30.1g carbohydrates, 4.8g fat, and 4g protein.

INGREDIENTS

1 cup basmati rice 1 teaspoon minced fresh ginger root 2 cups water 1 cup steamed vegetables

Carrots (about 3/4 cup) shredded

roasting peanuts (quarter cup)

depending on your personal preference

margarine (about 1 tbsp.

peppercorns to taste with cayenne pepper

chopped fresh cilantro and 1 onion, thinly sliced

DIRECTIONS

In a medium-sized saucepan, combine the rice and the water. Boil vigorously over high heat until the water is completely evaporated. Reduce the heat to low and cover the pan with a lid, allowing the vegetables to steam for about 20 minutes or until they are fork tender.

Meanwhile, grind the peanuts in a blender and set them aside while the rice is cooking. Medium heat should be used to warm up the margarine in a skillet. Toss in the onion and cook, stirring constantly, for about 10 minutes, or until the onion is soft and golden brown. Season with salt to taste after stirring in the ginger and carrots. Heat on low for 5 minutes, then cover with a lid. Combine the cayenne pepper and peanuts in a separate bowl and mix thoroughly. When the rice is finished cooking, pour it into the skillet and gently stir it to combine with the other components. Cilantro leaves can be used to garnish the dish.

BEETS 'N' SWEETS WITH ROASTING

| Prep time: 15 minutes | Cooking time: 1 hour 15 minutes

| Total time: 1 hour 15 minutes FACTS ABOUT VEGETABLE
NUTRITION

198 calories | 34.3 grams of carbohydrate | 5.9 grams of fat
| 3.5 grams of protein | 0 milligrams of cholesterol

INGREDIENTS

1 pound medium-sized beets, peeled and cut into chunks

black pepper (ground) 1 teaspoon

1/2 cup olive oil (divided into 2 1/2 tablespoons)

Sugar, 1 teaspoon (approximately).

1 teaspoon minced garlic (optional).

Cut 3 medium sweet potatoes into chunks (approximately).

1 teaspoon fine sea salt (kosher)

1 large sweet onion, peeled and finely minced

DIRECTIONS

Bake at 400 degrees Fahrenheit for 20 minutes (200 degrees
C).

Coat the beets with 1/2 tablespoon olive oil in a large mixing
bowl until they are well coated. On a baking sheet, spread the
mixture in a thin layer.

In a large resealable plastic bag, combine the remaining 2
tablespoons of olive oil, the garlic powder, the salt, the pepper,
and the sugar. Sweet potatoes and onion should be placed
in a bag for easy storage. Using a sealable bag, shake the
vegetables to evenly coat them in the oil mixture.

Beets should be baked for 15 minutes at 350°F. On a baking sheet, toss the sweet potato mixture with the beets. Continue to bake for another 45 minutes, stirring every 20 minutes, or until all vegetables are tender, stirring occasionally.

Chapter Two

A RED PEPPER HUMMUS WITH SPICED SWEET ROASTING

Preparation time: 15 minutes | Cooking time: 1 hour | Total time: 1h15 minutes | Time required for additional preparation is 15 minutes. FACTS ABOUT VEGETABLE NUTRITION

64 calories | 9.6 grams of carbohydrate | 2.2 grams of fat | 2.5 grams of protein | 0 milligrams of cholesterol

INGREDIENTS

Drain and rinse one (15-ounce) can garbanzo beans.

ground cumin (half a teaspoon)

roast red peppers, 1 (4-ounce) jar (4-ounce jar)

a half teaspoon of cayenne pepper (optional)

3 tablespoons lemon juice (or other citrus fruit juice)

salt (one-quarter teaspoon)

one-and-a-half tablespoons ground tahini

Fresh chopped parsley (about 1 teaspoon)

1 minced garlic clove (about 1 clove total)

DIRECTIONS

Puree the chickpeas, red peppers, lemon juice, tahini, garlic, cumin, cayenne pepper, and salt in an electric blender or food processor until smooth and creamy. Serve immediately. Mix until the mixture is fairly smooth and slightly fluffy, using long pulses to ensure that it doesn't become too thick. While processing or blending, make sure to scrape the mixture off the sides of the food processor or blender. Refrigerate for at least 1 hour after transferring to a serving bowl. (You can make the hummus up to 3 days ahead of time and store it in the refrigerator.) - Before serving, allow the dish to come to room temperature.

The chopped parsley should be sprinkled on top of the hummus before it is served.

POTATOES WITH SUGAR BAKED IN

Cooking time: 1 hour and 15 minutes | Preparation time: 10 minutes | Total time 1 hour and 15 minutes FACTS ABOUT VEGETABLE NUTRITION

321 calories | 61 grams of carbohydrate | 7.3 grams of fat | 4.8 grams of protein | 0 milligrams of cholesterol

INGREDIENTS

olive oil (about 2 tbsp.

3 large sweet potatoes, 2 pinches salt

black pepper, 2 pinches, freshly ground

oregano leaves (dried) 2 pinches

DIRECTIONS

350 degrees Fahrenheit for the oven (175 degrees C). Just enough olive oil to coat the bottom of a glass or nonstick baking dish will suffice.

The sweet potatoes should be washed and peeled. Reduce the size of the pieces to a medium size. Into a baking dish, place the sweet potatoes that have been cut into pieces and turn them to coat them with olive oil. Season with oregano, salt, and pepper to taste, but don't go overboard (to taste).

60 minutes or until the potatoes are soft in a preheated 350 degree F (175 degrees C) oven.

SPRING ROLLS IN VIETNAMESE CUISINE

Approximately 45 minutes to prepare, 5 minutes to cook, and 50 minutes to complete the entire recipe. FACTS ABOUT VEGETABLE NUTRITION

It contains: 82 calories, 15.7 grams of carbohydrates, 0.7 grams of fat, and 3.3 grams of protein. It has 11 milligrams of cholesterol.

INGREDIENTS

rice vermicelli (about 2 ounces)

one-fourth cup of distilled water

12 wrappers made of rice (8.5 inch diameter)

2 tbsp. lime juice (from fresh)

1 pound large cooked shrimp - peeled, deveined, and cut in half

1 minced garlic clove (about 1 clove total)

freshly chopped Thai basil (1 1/3 tablespoons)

sugar (white): 2 tablespoons

mint leaves, chopped (about 3 tablespoons), fresh

garlic chili sauce (1/2 teaspoon)

chopped fresh cilantro (about 3 tablespoons)

the hoisin sauce (three tablespoons)

2 lettuce leaves, finely minced

peanuts, chopped finely (1 teaspoon)

fish sauce (four teaspoons)

DIRECTIONS

Start by heating water in a medium-sized saucepan to a simmer. Cook the rice vermicelli for 3 to 5 minutes, or until al dente, and drain well afterwards.

A large bowl of warm water should be set aside for this project. Soften one wrapper by dipping it for one second into the hot water. Keep wrapper in a horizontal position. Place 2 shrimp halves, a handful of vermicelli, basil, mint, cilantro, and lettuce in a row across the center of the plate, leaving about 2 inches of space on each side. Repeat with the remaining ingredients. Using the lettuce as a starting point, start rolling from one end of the wrapper and working your way around it. Continually add ingredients until all are used.

Place all of the ingredients in a small bowl and stir well. Add the fish sauce and mix well.

Toss the hoisin sauce and peanuts together in a separate small bowl.

Combine the fish sauce and hoisin sauce mixtures and serve with the rolled spring rolls on a plate.

CURRY MADE WITH CHICKPEAS

| Prep time: 10 minutes | Cooking time: 30 minutes | Total time: 40 minutes | 8 servings FACTS ABOUT VEGETABLE NUTRITION

135 calories | 20.5 grams of carbohydrate | 4.5 grams of fat | 4.1 grams of protein | 0 milligrams of cholesterol

INGREDIENTS

vegetable oil (about 2 tbsp.)

coriander leaves (ground) 1 teaspoon

Salt and pepper to taste 2 onions, minced

garlic, minced (about 2 cloves total)

Cayenne pepper, 1 teaspoon 2 teaspoons finely chopped fresh ginger root,

Turmeric powder (1 teaspoon)

6 cloves that are whole

Can of garbanzo beans (approximately 15-ounce size)

2 (2-inch) cinnamon sticks, finely ground

1 cup fresh cilantro, finely minced.

1 teaspoon cumin seeds (ground)

DIRECTIONS

Over medium heat, heat oil in a large frying pan and cook onions until tender, stirring occasionally.

Using a large mixing bowl, combine the ingredients for the garlic ginger cloves cinnamon cumin coriander salt cayenne pepper and turmeric in a whirl. Using a constant stream of stirring, cook for 1 minute over medium heat. Toss in the garbanzo beans as well as any liquid. Continually cook, stirring constantly, until all of the ingredients are well combined and thoroughly warmed. Take the pan off the stovetop and put it somewhere safe to cool. Remove 1 tablespoon of the cilantro for garnish and stir it in just before serving. DIRECTIONS:

POTATOES ON THE COOKER GRILL

Prepare for four servings in ten minutes, cook for twenty minutes, and cook for the entire thirty minutes. FACTS ABOUT VEGETABLE NUTRITION

227 calories | 36.4 grams of carbohydrate | 7.3 grams of fat | 4.3 grams of protein | 0 milligrams of cholesterol

INGREDIENTS

2 lbs red potatoes, quartered 2 lbs sweet potatoes peppercorns that have been freshly ground vegetable oil (about 2 tbsp.)
a half teaspoon of dried rosemary, ground
Salt (about 1 teaspoon)

DIRECTIONS

Bake at 450 degrees Fahrenheit for 15 minutes until golden brown (250 degrees C).

Toss the potatoes in a large roasting pan with the oil, salt, pepper, and rosemary until they are evenly coated. Make a single layer of potatoes and spread them out on the baking sheet.

Cook for 20 minutes, stirring occasionally, in the preheated oven. Serve as soon as possible after preparing it.

BEANS IN THE OVEN

| Prep time: 20 minutes | Cooking time: 1 hour and 20 minutes | Total time: 1h20 minutes | 6 servings FACTS ABOUT VEGETABLE NUTRITION

287 calories | 52.3 grams of carbohydrate | 6.5 grams of fat | 8.9 grams of protein | 16 milligrams of cholesterol

INGREDIENTS

1 tin (15 ounces) baked beans with bacon
tablespoon Worcestershire sauce (optional)
brown sugar that has been sealed in a jar
1 tablespoon red wine vinegar (optional)
salt and pepper to taste; 1/2 onion, chopped
half-cup ketchup (or other condiment)
Bacon (two slices)
prepared mustard (about 1 tbsp.

DIRECTIONS

350 degrees Fahrenheit for the oven (175 degrees C).

Using a 9-by-9-inch baking dish, combine the pork and beans with the brown sugar, onion, ketchup, mustard, Worcestershire sauce, vinegar, and salt and pepper to taste in a large mixing bowl. The bacon slices should be placed on top.

350 degrees F (175 degrees C) for 1 hour, or until sauce has thickened and bacon has been cooked, whichever comes first.

AMATRICIANA

Approximately 35 minutes total time: 15 minutes for preparation, 20 minutes for cooking. FACTS ABOUT VEGETABLE NUTRITION

Amount per serving: 529 calories | 97.6 grams of carbohydrates | 7.5 grams of fat | 21 grams of protein | 12 milligrams of cholesterol

INGREDIENTS

two (15 ounce) cans stewed tomatoes, diced 4 slices bacon, diced

onion, chopped (about 1/2 cup)

pasta (uncooked): 1 pound linguine

1 teaspoon minced garlic, preferably fresh.

freshly chopped basil (about 1 tablespoon total)

red pepper flakes (crushed) 1/4 teaspoon

2 tbsp. grated Parmesan cheese (optional).

DIRECTIONS

Sauté the diced bacon in a large saucepan over medium-high heat for 5 minutes or until it is crisp, stirring occasionally. Remove all of the drippings from the pan except for 2 tablespoons and set aside.

Cook for about 3 minutes over medium heat, until the onions have softened slightly. Cook for 30 seconds after incorporating the garlic and red pepper flakes. Cook for 10 minutes, breaking up the tomatoes, after which remove from heat.

During this time, cook the pasta in a large pot of boiling salted water until al dente in a large pot of salted water. Drain.

Toss the cooked pasta with the sauce after it has been stirred in. Grated Parmesan cheese should be sprinkled on top.

RED BEANS AND RICE ARE SIMPLE TO MAKE.

| Prep time: 10 minutes | Cooking time: 30 minutes | Total time: 40 minutes | 8 servings FACTS ABOUT VEGETABLE NUTRITION

289 calories | 42.4 grams of carbohydrate | 5.7 grams of fat | 16.3 grams of protein | 35 milligrams of cholesterol

INGREDIENTS

Water (two cups)

canned kidney beans, drained from 2 (15-ounce cans)

2 cups rice that hasn't been cooked

12 ounce whole peeled tomatoes, chopped 1 pound turkey kielbasa, cut diagonally into 1/4 inch slices 1 pound whole peeled tomatoes, diced

oregano leaves (about 1/2 teaspoon)

2 cloves of garlic, finely chopped, salt and pepper

half a teaspoon of freshly ground pepper 1 green onion, chopped

Garlic, minced (one clove)

DIRECTIONS

Cooking liquid comes to a boil in a saucepan. Stir in the rice until it is well-combined. Cover and cook for another 20 minutes on low heat.

Sauté the sausage for 5 minutes in a large skillet over low heat. Continue to saute until the vegetables are tender, about

10 minutes. Place beans and tomatoes in a large mixing bowl with juice added. Add oregano, salt, and pepper to taste and season to your liking. 20 minutes should be enough time to cook the vegetables uncovered. Toss with rice and enjoy!

DEL GALLO (Picture of the Galloway)

Servings: 12 | Prep time: 20 minutes | Cooking time: 3 hours | Total time: 3 hours and 20 minutes | Extra time: 3 hours and 20 minutes COMPLETE NUTRITION FACTS Calories: 10 | Carbohydrates: 2.2g | Fat: 0.1g | Protein: 0.4g | Cholesterol: 0mg |

INGREDIENTS

1 cup diced roma (plum) tomatoes

1 minced garlic clove (about 1 clove total)

finely chopped half a red onion

Garlic powder (about 1 teaspoon)

chopped fresh cilantro (about 3 tablespoons)

or to taste, 1 teaspoon ground cumin

half a jalapeno pepper, seeded and minced with salt and freshly ground black pepper to taste.

Lime juice from half a lime

DIRECTIONS 1. In a large mixing bowl, combine the tomatoes, onion, cilantro, jalapeno pepper, lime juice, garlic, garlic powder, cumin, salt, and pepper. Preparation time: Refrigerate for at least 3 hours before serving

YAKISOBA CHICKEN is a Japanese dish that consists of chicken, rice, and vegetables.

Making 6 servings will take approximately 15 minutes of preparation, 15 minutes of cooking, and 30 minutes total.

FACTS ABOUT VEGETABLE NUTRITION

295 calories | 40.7 grams of carbohydrate | 4.8 grams of fat | 26.3 grams of protein | 46 milligrams of cholesterol

INGREDIENTS

a half teaspoon of sesame seed oil

Soy sauce (1/2 cup)

canola oil (about 1 tbsp.

1-inch piece of onion, sliced crosswise into eighths

chili paste (about 2 tbsp.)

cabbage, roughly chopped (half a medium head)

Garlic (two cloves, chopped) and carrots (two carrots, coarsely chopped)

Cubes of chicken breast, skinless and boneless, cut into four 1-inch pieces

Cooked and drained soba noodles (eight ounces).

DIRECTIONS

Cook for 30 seconds in a large skillet with sesame oil, canola oil, garlic, and chili paste. Add the garlic and cook for another 30 seconds, stirring constantly. Stir-fry for 5 minutes, or until the chicken is no longer pink, with 1/4 cup soy sauce, until the sauce has thickened. Keep warm by removing the mixture from the pan and placing it in a separate bowl.

Combine the onion, cabbage, and carrots in the pan that has been empty for a while now. Stir-fry for 2 to 3 minutes, or until cabbage starts to wilt. In a separate pan, heat the remaining soy sauce until it is hot. Add the cooked noodles and chicken mixture to the pan and mix well. Prepare the dish and serve it to your friends.

FOOD CAKE IN THE SHADOWS

| Prep time: 30 minutes | Cooking time: 45 minutes | Total time: 1h15 minutes | 14 servings FACTS ABOUT VEGETABLE NUTRITION

Amount per serving: 136 calories | 20.9 grams of carbohydrates | 0.1 grams of fat | 4 grams of protein | zero milligrams of cholesterol

INGREDIENTS

Cake flour 1 1/2 teaspoons vanilla extract 1.5 cups white sugar 2 tablespoons melted butter

cream of tartar (1 1/2 teaspoons)

Egg whites (a total of twelve)

salt (half a teaspoon)

DIRECTIONS

Prepare your baking sheet by preheating the oven to 375°F. Prepare your 10 inch tube pan by wiping it down with a clean, dry cloth. If there is any oil or residue present, the egg whites will deflate quickly. Set aside the flour and 3/4 cup of the sugar that you sifted together earlier in the process.

Set aside a large mixing bowl and whisk it constantly until the egg whites are medium stiff peaks. Fold in the vanilla extract, cream of tartar, and salt. Whip the mixture until stiff peaks are formed, gradually adding the remaining sugar. As soon as the egg white mixture has reached its maximum volume, begin folding in the sifted ingredients in thirds, beginning with the first third. Overmixing is not allowed. Fill the tube pan halfway with the batter and bake for 30 minutes.

Bake in the preheated oven for 40 to 45 minutes, or until the cake springs back when lightly touched. In order to prevent decompression while cooling, the tube pan should be balanced upside down on the top of a bottle, as shown. Run a knife around the edge of the pan and invert the pan onto a plate when the pan has cooled completely.

SALAD WITH MANGOES

| Prep time: 15 minutes | Cooking time: 30 minutes | Total time: 45 minutes | Additional preparation time of 30 minutes

NUTRITIONAL FACTS: Calories: 21 | Carbohydrates: 5.4g | Fat: 0.1g | Protein: 0.3g | Cholesterol: 0mg |

INGREDIENTS

1 mango - peeled, seeded, and chopped (optional).

1/2 cup finely chopped fresh jalapeno chile peppers

1/4 cup red bell pepper, finely chopped

Lime juice, 2 tablespoons

1 green onion, peeled and finely minced

Lemon juice (about 1 tablespoon)

chopped cilantro (about 2 tablespoons)

Instructions 1. In a medium-sized mixing bowl, combine mango, red bell pepper, green onion, cilantro, jalapeno, lime juice, and lemon juice until well combined. Allow at least 30 minutes to pass before serving after covering with plastic wrap.

WITH SECRET HOBO SPICES, BLACKENED TILAPIA

| Prep time: 10 minutes | Cooking time: 8 minutes | Total time: 18 minutes | 4 servings THE NUTRITION INFORMATION Calories: 245 | Carbohydrates: 21.5g | Fat: 6.8g | Protein: 26.8g | Cholesterol: 42 mg

INGREDIENTS

1 cup paprika, chopped

1 teaspoon thyme leaves, dried

onion powder (about 1 tablespoon)

celery seed (1/2 teaspoon)

Garlic powder (about 1 teaspoon)

or to your liking, 1 tablespoon kosher salt

peppercorns, ground (about a teaspoon worth)

Tilapia fillets (about 1 pound total)

black pepper (ground) 1 teaspoon

2 wedges of lemon, cut into quarters

or to your personal preference, 1 teaspoon cayenne pepper

White bread (four slices)

dried oregano (1 teaspoon)

1/4 cup lard or other cooking fat

DIRECTIONS

The spice blend should be prepared in a small bowl or jar with a tight-fitting lid. Combine the paprika, onion powder, garlic powder, white pepper, black pepper, cayenne pepper, oregano, thyme, celery seed, and kosher salt in a large mixing bowl until well combined. Allow the fish fillets to rest at room temperature for no more than 30 minutes after being coated with the spice mixture.

Heat a heavy skillet over high heat. Add oil, and heat until it is almost smoking. Place the fillets in the pan, and cook for about 3 minutes per side, or until fish is opaque and can be flaked with a fork. Remove from the pan, and place onto slices of white bread. Pour pan juices over them and squeeze lemon juice all over. Do not underestimate the white bread. It gets quite tasty soaking up all the juices.

Chapter Three

PERFECT SUSHI RICE

Servings: 15 | Prep: 5m | Cooks: 20m | Total: 25m FACTS ABOUT VEGETABLE NUTRITION

Calories: 112 | Carbohydrates: 23.5g | Fat: 1g | Protein: 1.7g | Cholesterol: 0mg

INGREDIENTS

2 cups uncooked glutinous white rice (sushi rice) (sushi rice)

1/4 cup lard or other cooking fat

3 cups water

1/4 cup white sugar

1/2 cup rice vinegar

Salt (about 1 teaspoon)

DIRECTIONS

Rinse the rice in a strainer or colander until the water runs clear. Combine with water in a medium saucepan. Bring to a boil, then reduce the heat to low, cover and cook for 20 minutes. Rice should be tender and water should be absorbed. Cool until cool enough to handle.

In a small saucepan, combine the rice vinegar, oil, sugar and salt. Cook over medium heat until the sugar dissolves. Cool, then stir into the cooked rice. When you pour this in to the rice it will seem very wet. Keep stirring and the rice will dry as it cools.

SALAD WITH MANGOES

| Prep time: 15 minutes | Cooking time: 30 minutes | Total time: 45 minutes | Additional preparation time of 30 minutes NUTRITION FACTS\sCalories: 21 | Carbohydrates: 5.4g | Fat: 0.1g | Protein: 0.3g | Cholesterol: 0mg

INGREDIENTS

1 mango - peeled, seeded, and chopped (optional).

1/2 cup finely chopped fresh jalapeno chile peppers

1/4 cup red bell pepper, finely chopped

Lime juice, 2 tablespoons

1 green onion, peeled and finely minced

Lemon juice (about 1 tablespoon)

chopped cilantro (about 2 tablespoons)

Instructions 1. In a medium-sized mixing bowl, combine mango, red bell pepper, green onion, cilantro, jalapeno, lime juice, and lemon juice until well combined. Allow at least 30 minutes to pass before serving after covering with plastic wrap.

MOROCCAN-STYLE STUFFED ACORN SQUASH

Servings: 4 | Prep: 15m | Cooks: 45m | Total: 1h NUTRITION FACTS\sCalories: 502 | Carbohydrates: 93.8g | Fat: 11.7g | Protein: 11.2g | Cholesterol: 10mg

INGREDIENTS

2 tablespoons brown sugar

1 cup garbanzo beans, drained

1 tablespoon butter, melted

1/2 cup raisins

2 large acorn squash, halved and seeded

1 1/2 tablespoons ground cumin

2 tablespoons olive oil\ssalt and pepper to taste

2 cloves garlic, chopped

1 (14 ounce) can chicken broth

2 stalks celery, chopped

1 cup uncooked couscous

2 carrots, chopped

DIRECTIONS

350 degrees Fahrenheit for the oven (175 degrees C).

Arrange squash halves cut side down on a baking sheet. Bake 30 minutes, or until tender. Dissolve the sugar in the melted butter. Brush squash with the butter mixture, and keep squash warm while preparing the stuffing.

Heat the olive oil in a skillet over medium heat. Stir in the garlic, celery, and carrots, and cook 5 minutes. Mix in the garbanzo beans and raisins. Season with cumin, salt, and pepper, and continue to cook and stir until vegetables are tender.

Pour the chicken broth into the skillet, and mix in the couscous. Cover skillet, and turn off heat. Allow couscous to absorb liquid for 5 minutes. Stuff squash halves with the skillet mixture to serve.

HONEY GARLIC CHICKEN IN THE SLOW COOKER

Prepare: 20 minutes; cook: 4 hours and 20 minutes; total preparation and preparation: 4 hours and 20 minutes. FACTS ABOUT VEGETABLE NUTRITION

235 calories | 34.4 grams of carbohydrate | 6 grams of fat | 13 grams of protein | 42 milligrams of cholesterol

INGREDIENTS

1/4 cup lard or other cooking fat

8-10 boneless thighs of chicken (without skin) with 2 garlic cloves smashed

Fresh ginger root, roughly chopped (about 1 tablespoon)

3/4 cup honey (optional).

2 – 20 ounce can of pineapple tidbits, drained but with liquid saved

Soy sauce (light) - 3/4 cup

cornstarch (about 2 tablespoons)

1 cup ketchup (optional)

one-fourth cup of distilled water

DIRECTIONS

Cook the chicken thighs in a pan over medium heat until they are uniformly browned on both sides, about 3 minutes per side total. In a slow cooker, place the chicken thighs.

In a large mixing bowl, combine the honey, soy sauce, ketchup, garlic, ginger, and pineapple juice that has been set aside for serving. Into the slow cooker, add the other ingredients and stir.

On high, cook for four hours, covered. Just before serving, add the pineapple tidbits.

In a small bowl, whisk together the cornstarch and water. Turn off the slow cooker and set it aside to cool. Cook on low for 4 hours or on high for 6 hours. Stir in cornstarch mixture to leftover sauce. Toss the chicken with the sauce and serve.

COOKED APPLESAUCE WITH SPICES IN THE SLOW COOKER

6 hours and 40 minutes to prepare 8 servings, cook for 6 hours and 30 minutes, then clean up after yourself. FACTS ABOUT VEGETABLE NUTRITION

Nutrition facts: 150 calories, 39.4 grams of carbohydrates, 0.2 gram of fat, 0.4 grams of protein, and zero milligrams of cholesterol

INGREDIENTS

6 to 8 apples (peeled, cored, and thinly sliced).

7/32 cup brown sugar that has been packed

water (half a cup)

pumpkin pie spice (1/2 teaspoon)

DIRECTIONS 1. In a slow cooker, combine the apples and water; simmer on Low for 6 to 8 hours or until the apples are soft. Cook for a further 30 minutes after adding the brown sugar and pumpkin pie spice.

KALE FROM THE MEDIEVAL

Cooking Time: 10 Minutes | Total Time: 25 Minutes | Servings: 6 FACTS ABOUT VEGETABLE NUTRITION

91 calories | 14.5 grams of carbohydrate | 3.2 grams of fat | 4.6 grams of protein | 0 milligrams of cholesterol

INGREDIENTS

10 to 12 cups of kale, roughly chopped

soy sauce (1 teaspoon)

Lemon juice (about 2 tbsp.

depending on your own preference

1-tablespoon extra-virgin olive oil, or more to taste if necessary; freshly ground black pepper

1 tablespoon minced garlic, preferably fresh.

DIRECTIONS

To steam vegetables, place a steamer insert into a saucepan and fill with water to just below the steamer's base. Cover the pan and bring the water to a boil over high heat, stirring occasionally.. Add the kale and cover with a lid, steaming until barely soft, 7 to 10 minutes, depending on thickness of kale leaves.

Combine the lemon juice, olive oil, garlic, soy sauce and salt & pepper in a large mixing bowl until well-combined and well-seasoned. Using your hands, thoroughly coat the kale with the dressing.

SPRING PASTA WITH SCALLOPS, ZUCCHINI, AND TOMATOES

| Prep time: 15 minutes | Cooking time: 15 minutes | Total time: 30 minutes 8 servings Nutritional Information: 335 calories | 46.1 grams of carbohydrate | 9.1 grams of fat | 18.7 grams of protein | 20 milligrams of cholesterol

INGREDIENTS

2 tablespoons crushed red pepper flakes 1 pound dried fettuccine pasta

4 tablespoons extra-virgin olive oil

basil leaves (chopped) 1 cup

minced 4 roma (plum) tomatoes, 2 zucchinis, diced 1 onion 3 garlic cloves, minced

Bay scallops weighing 1 pound

a half teaspoon of salt and two tablespoons of grated Parmesan

DIRECTIONS

Cook the pasta till al dente in a big pot of boiling salted water. Drain.

Between times, heat the oil in a big pan and sauté the garlic until soft. Continue to sauté for 10 minutes while adding salt, red pepper flakes, and dried basil, if using. Continue to cook for another 5 minutes, or until the scallops are opaque. Add the chopped tomatoes, bay scallops, and fresh basil, if desired.

Cooked pasta should be poured over the sauce, which should be garnished with grated Parmesan.

SERVINGS: 4 | PREP TIME: 15 M | COOK TIME: 25 M | TOTAL TIME: 40 MONEY PER SERVING Nutrient Facts: 450 calories | 67.1 grams of carbohydrates | 14.9 grams of fat | 16.5 grams of protein | 2 milligrams of cholesterol

INGREDIENTS

olive oil (around 1 tablespoon)

red pepper flakes (or to taste) 1 tablespoon

1 jalapeño pepper, peeled and finely minced

1 1/2 teaspoons cayenne pepper powder

2 garlic cloves, peeled and minced

cumin powder (1/2 teaspoon)

black beans (1 (15 ounce can), washed and drained 1 (15 ounce can of black beans

Taste and season with 1 teaspoon of kosher salt and freshly ground black pepper

fire-roasted diced tomatoes, 1 (14.5 ounce) can

1. 1 avocado - peeled, pitted, and chopped

1 cup yellow corn (or any similar sized quantity)

Lime juiced to a desired consistency

quinoa (one cup)

cilantro, 2 teaspoons finely chopped

broth (chicken or vegetable) 1 cup

DIRECTIONS

Over medium-high heat, warm the oil in a large skillet. Using heated oil, saute the jalapeño pepper and garlic for approximately 1 minute, or until they become aromatic.

Then add the red pepper flakes and season with salt and pepper to taste. Add the black beans, tomatoes, yellow corn, and chicken broth to the pan and stir until everything is well-combined. Simmer for approximately 20 minutes, after which you should cover the pan with a lid and turn the heat down to low to ensure that the quinoa is cooked and all of the liquid has been absorbed. In a large mixing bowl, blend avocado, lime juice, and cilantro until well incorporated. quinoa

BAKED SWEET POTATO IN A CAJUN STYLE.

| Prep time: 10 minutes | Cooking time: 1 hour and 10 minutes | Total preparation time: 1h10 minutes. FACTS ABOUT VEGETABLE NUTRITION

Amount per serving: 229 calories | 49.1 grams of carbohydrates | 2.3 grams of fat | 4.8 grams of protein

INGREDIENTS

1/4 cup paprika, 1/2 teaspoon cumin

1/4 teaspoon ground rosemary (optional)

sugar (brown): 1 teaspoon

garlic powder (one-fourth teaspoon)

black pepper (around 1/4 teaspoon)

cayenne pepper, 1/8 teaspoon

onion powder (quarter teaspoon)

sweet potatoes (around 2 lbs)

1 1/2 tablespoons extra-virgin olive oil 1/4 teaspoon fresh thyme

DIRECTIONS

Oven should be preheated at 375 degrees Fahrenheit (190 degrees C).

Toss together paprika, brown sugar, black pepper, onion powder, thyme and rosemary, garlic powder, and cayenne pepper in a small mixing bowl until evenly combined.

Make a cut through the middle of the sweet potatoes lengthwise. Olive oil should be brushed across both halves. Season the cut surfaces of each half with the seasoning mixture. Using a baking sheet or a small pan, spread out the sweet potatoes.

Baking for around 1 hour in a preheated oven will provide a tender result.

PORK CHOPS WITH A SPICY PEACH GLAZING

Prepare for four servings in ten minutes, cook for twenty minutes, then cook for the whole thirty minutes. Nutritional Facts: 404 calories | 58.2 grams of carbohydrates | 11.5 grams of fat | 13.2 grams of protein | 36 milligrams of cholesterol

INGREDIENTS

one-and-a-half cups peach jam

ground cinnamon (about 1 pinch)

15 tablespoons Worcestershire sauce, to taste (with salt and pepper).

chili paste (half a teaspoon)

vegetable oil (around 2 tbsp.)

pork chops (without bones) 4 lbs.

white wine (1/2 cup)

ground ginger (one teaspoon)

DIRECTIONS

Combine the peach preserves, Worcestershire sauce, and chile paste in a small mixing bowl until well blended. Clean and pat dry the pork chops. Season the chops with ginger, cinnamon, salt, and pepper to taste before serving them up.

Over medium-high heat, warm the oil in a large skillet. The chops should be seared for about 2 minutes each side. Toss out of the pan and place on a plate to cool.

In a small saucepan, add the white wine and whisk to scrape up any browned bits from the bottom. Combine the peach preserves and the other ingredients. Stir until everything is well combined. To finish, return the chops to the pan and turn to coat them with the sauce on both sides. Reduce the heat to medium-low and cook the pork chops for about 8 minutes on each side, or until they are cooked to your satisfaction.

REAL FRENCH MERINGUES MADE WITHOUT CHEATING

| Preparation: 20 minutes | Cooking: 3 hours and 20 minutes | Total Time (3 hours and 20 minutes) | COMPLETE NUTRITION FACTS Calories: 31; Carbohydrates: 7.5g; Fat: 0g; Protein: 0.4g; Cholesterol: 0 mg

INGREDIENTS

confectioners' sugar (about 2 1/4 cups) 4 egg whites

DIRECTIONS

200 degrees Fahrenheit should be set in the oven (95 degrees C). A baking sheet should be greased and dusted with flour.

Make egg whites frothy in a glass or metal mixing bowl by using an electric mixer on high speed until stiff peaks form. While continuing to beat at medium speed, gradually add the sugar, a little at a time. Stop mixing until the mixture becomes firm and glossy, like satin, and transfer the mixture to a large pastry bag to finish piping the mixture. Using a big round tip or a star tip, pipe the meringue onto the baking sheet that has been prepped.

In order to prevent the oven door from shutting completely, insert a wooden spoon handle in the oven and close the door. Allow meringues to bake for 3 hours, or until they are dry and can be easily removed from the pan. Before keeping cookies in an airtight container at room temperature, allow them to cool fully.

DESSERT WITH BAKED FRENCH FRIED TOMATOES

Approximately 45 minutes total time: 20 minutes for preparation, 25 minutes for cooking. FACTS ABOUT VEGETABLE NUTRITION

140 calories, 28.2 grams of carbs, 1.5 grams of fat, five grams of protein, and four milligrams of cholesterol.

INGREDIENTS

3 russet potatoes, quartered and cut into 1/4-inch wide strips.

cooking spray, salt, and pepper to taste 1/4 cup grated Parmesan cheese

1 tbsp. dry basil, chopped

DIRECTIONS

Bake at 400 degrees Fahrenheit for 20 minutes (200 degrees C). A medium baking sheet should be lightly greased.

Potato strips should be arranged in a single layer on the baking sheet that has been prepared, skin side up. Season with basil, Parmesan cheese, salt, and pepper after gently spraying with cooking spray.

25 minutes or until the top is golden brown in a preheated oven at 350°F (180°C).

ASPARAGUS THAT MOVES QUICKLY

| Prep time: 5 minutes | Cooking time: 10 minutes | Total time: 15 minutes | FACTS ABOUT VEGETABLE NUTRITION

Amount per serving: 32 calories | 6.3 grams of carbohydrates | 0.2 grams of fat | 3.4 grams of protein | zero milligrams of cholesterol

INGREDIENTS

one-half cup Cajun seasoning 1 pound asparagus

DIRECTIONS

425 degrees Fahrenheit should be set for the oven (220 degrees C).

Using the sensitive section of the asparagus stem, snap off the asparagus. Distribute the spears on a baking sheet so that they are all on the same layer. Cajun spice should be sparingly sprayed on after you have sprayed with the nonstick spray.

10 minutes or until the vegetables are soft in the preheated oven.

Chapter Four

THE PASTA FROM MEXICO.

| Prep time: 5 minutes | Cooking time: 15 minutes |
Total time: 20 minutes 4 servings FACTS ABOUT VEGETABLE
NUTRITION

358 calories | 59.5 grams of carbohydrate | 9.4 grams of fat
| 10.3 grams of protein | 0 milligrams of cholesterol
INGREDIENTS

Seashell pasta (1/2 pound):

peeled and chopped tomatoes from a 14.5-ounce can 1

olive oil (around 2 tbsp.

salsa (a quarter cup)

cut up 2 onions (see recipe below)

black olives (sliced) 1/4 cup

2 tablespoons finely minced green bell pepper

1/4 cup taco seasoning mix (optional)

Sweet corn kernels (about half a cup).

to taste with salt and pepper

black beans (one can, 15 ounces), drained

DIRECTIONS

Start by filling a big saucepan halfway with lightly salted water and bringing it to a boil. Cook the pasta for 8 to 10 minutes, or until it is al dente, before draining it from the water.

Meanwhile, heat the olive oil in a big pan over medium heat, while the pasta is cooking (about 10 minutes). Sauté the onions and peppers in the oil for about 10 minutes, or until they are gently browned. Continue to heat until corn is fully incorporated. Cook for 5 minutes, stirring often, until the black beans, tomatoes, salsa, olives, taco seasoning, salt, and pepper are well heated.

Prepare pasta according to package directions.

SALAD ORIGINAL

Preparation time: 20 minutes | Cooking time: 15 minutes | Total time: 35 minutes | 48 servings FACTS ABOUT VEGETABLE NUTRITION

The following are the nutritional values: 6 calories, 1.5 grams of carbohydrates, 0 grams of fat, 0.2 grams of protein, and zero milligrams of cholesterol.

INGREDIENTS

4 chile peppers (jalapenos) smashed

5 garlic cloves, coarsely sliced 1 teaspoon salt 1 teaspoon sugar

ground cumin (1/4 teaspoon)

cut finely 1 medium onion (optional)

2 chopped tomatoes with green chile peppers from a 10-ounce can

sugar (white) - 1 tablespoon

entire peeled tomatoes from a can (28 ounces).

DIRECTIONS

Bake at 400 degrees Fahrenheit for 20 minutes (200 degrees C).

On a medium baking sheet, arrange the jalapeño chile peppers. Bake for 15 minutes or until the vegetables are roasted in the preheated oven. Using tongs, carefully remove stems from the pan.

Using a blender or food processor, puree the jalapeño chile peppers with the garlic and onion. Add the white sugar and salt to taste. Add the diced tomatoes with green chile peppers. Chop for a few seconds while using the pulse function. Whole peeled tomatoes should be added at this point as a finishing touch. Chop until desired consistency is achieved by using the pulse setting. Toss the ingredients into a medium-sized mixing basin. Refrigerate until ready to serve by covering with plastic wrap.

VEGETABLE MEDLEY WITH ROASTED VEGETABLE

Making 6 servings will take 25 minutes prep time, 1 hour cooking time, a total of 1 hour 55 minutes, and an additional 30 minutes. FACTS ABOUT VEGETABLE NUTRITION

There are 192 calories in this recipe. There are 34.6 gram of carbohydrates, 5 grams of fat, 4 grams of protein, and 0 milligrams of cholesterol.

INGREDIENTS

Divide the olive oil into two equal halves.

cut into 1-inch slices half a cup roasted red peppers

1 giant yam, peeled and sliced into 1-inch chunks.

garlic, minced (about 2 cloves total)

1 big parsnip, peeled and sliced into 1 inch chunks (or smaller).

freshly chopped basil (about a quarter cup)

Baby carrots (about 1 cup)

salt (kosher) to taste (1/2 teaspoon)

1 zucchini, peeled and sliced into 1-inch thick slices.

peppercorns, 1/2 teaspoon freshly ground

1 bunch of fresh asparagus, trimmed and sliced into 1-inch-thick slices

DIRECTIONS

425 degrees Fahrenheit should be set for the oven (220 degrees C). 1 tablespoon olive oil should be used to grease 2 baking sheets.

Place the yams, parsnips, and carrots on the baking pans and bake for 30 minutes at 350 degrees. Place the zucchini and asparagus in the preheated oven for 30 minutes, then sprinkle with the remaining 1 tablespoon of olive oil and bake for another 15 minutes. Continue baking for another 30 minutes or until all of the veggies are soft. Removing the baking sheet from the oven and allowing it to cool for 30 minutes will ensure that the potatoes are cooked through and tender.

In a large mixing bowl, toss the roasted peppers with the garlic, basil, salt, and pepper until everything is well-combined and evenly distributed. In a large mixing bowl, combine the roasted veggies. Room temperature or chilled are both acceptable serving temperatures.

MEAT PASTA WITH ASPARAGUS, CHICKEN, AND PENE

| Prep time: 15 minutes | Cooking time: 20 minutes | Total time: 35 minutes | 8 servings 311 calories | 43.2 grams of carbohydrates | 6.8 grams of fat | 20.3 grams of protein | Cholesterol 29 milligrams

INGREDIENTS

Dry penne pasta (about 16 ounces)

Cut 12 ounces of asparagus into 1 inch pieces after trimming and dicing it.

Divide the olive oil into two equal halves.

1-teaspoon red pepper flakes that have been crushed

3/4 pound skinless, boneless chicken breast flesh - cut into bite-size pieces; season with salt and pepper to taste.

garlic, minced (four cloves)

Parmesan cheese, 1/2 cup grated

DIRECTIONS

Start by filling a big saucepan halfway with lightly salted water and bringing it to a boil. Cook the pasta for 8 to 10 minutes, or until it is al dente, in a pot of boiling salted water. Place in a large mixing bowl after draining.

Large skillet over medium heat with 1 tablespoon olive oil, 1 tablespoon butter, 1 tablespoon salt, 1 tablespoon pepper Remove the chicken from the pan after it has become firm and lightly browned. Add the remaining tablespoon of olive oil to the skillet and stir to combine the flavors. Continue to cook and stir the garlic, asparagus, and red pepper flakes in the oil until the asparagus is tender. Cook for 2 minutes, stirring frequently, to ensure that the flavors are well blended. Sea salt and freshly ground pepper are added for seasoning.

Combination of chicken and asparagus should be tossed into a pasta dish. Parmesan cheese is sprinkled on top.

FAJITAS ARE AMAZING

| Prep time: 15 minutes | Cooking time: 15 minutes | Total time: 30 minutes | Servings: 10 FACTS ABOUT VEGETABLE NUTRITION

427 calories | 64.2 grams of carbohydrate | 10.3 grams of fat | 18 grams of protein | 21 milligrams of cholesterol

INGREDIENTS

2-inch-thick slices of green bell pepper

cooked chicken meat (diced) 2 cups

7-ounce package dry Italian-style salad dressing (1 red bell pepper, sliced) 1 red onion, sliced mix

8 tortillas (12 inch diameter) made with 1 onion, thinly sliced mushrooms, 1 cup, freshly sliced

DIRECTIONS

Peppers and onions should be thinly sliced for this recipe. Slices should be long and thin, not diced.

To make the peppers and onion tender, saute them in a small amount of oil. Mushrooms and chicken should be added at this point. Maintain a low heat until the dish is completely heated. Completely incorporate the dry salad dressing mixture.

Pre-heat the tortillas and stuff them with the mixture. If desired, add shredded cheddar cheese, diced tomato, and shredded lettuce to the top of the sandwich..

Mexican Rice from MARIA'S RESTAURANT.

Cooking Time: 30 Minutes | Total Time: 40 Minutes | Servings: 6 FACTS ABOUT VEGETABLE NUTRITION

Nutritious and filling, with only 164 calories and 26.8 grams of carbohydrate, fat (4.9 grams), and protein (2.7 grams).

INGREDIENTS

olive oil (around 2 tbsp.

1 cup cooked brown rice 1/8 teaspoon freshly ground pepper

1.5 cups water 1 large onion, diced 2 1/2 cups water

Tomato sauce (one-third cup)

1 tablespoon chicken bouillon 1 1/2 teaspoons salt (such as Knorr)

1 serrano chile pepper (whole) 1/8 teaspoon ground cumin (optional)

1. In a medium-sized saucepan, heat the oil over medium heat until shimmering. Add salt, cumin, and pepper to taste and continue cooking and stirring until the rice and onion are browned, about 5 minutes. In a separate bowl, combine the rice and water. Water should be flavored with tomato sauce and chicken bouillon. Cook over medium-high heat until the water comes to a boil, then remove the saucepan's lid. Cook for another 10 minutes at a boil after adding the serrano chile pepper. Heat on medium-low for 15 to 20 minutes longer, or until the rice is tender and the water has been absorbed.

THE LINGUINE WITH PEPPERED BACON AND TOMATO

Making 6 servings will take approximately 15 minutes of preparation, 15 minutes of cooking, and 30 minutes total. Nutritional Information: 362 calories; 57.5 grams of carbohydrates; 7.6 grams of fat; 16.2 grams of protein; 16 milligrams of cholesterol

INGREDIENTS

peppered bacon, diced (1/2 pound total)

1 teaspoon sea salt 2 tablespoons finely chopped green onion freshly ground black pepper to your preference

minced garlic, 2 teaspoons

2 packages (each containing 16 ounces) linguine

Tomatoes, diced, from a 14.5-ounce can

Parmesan cheese (about 3 tablespoons)

1 tbsp. dry basil, chopped

DIRECTIONS

A large, deep skillet is ideal for cooking bacon. Continue to cook until evenly browned over medium-high heat. Pour off the liquid, reserving the drippings.

Cook the green onion and garlic for one minute in the bacon drippings on medium heat. Continue to cook for 5 minutes after adding the tomatoes and basil and seasonings.

Prepare a large pot of lightly salted water to boil in the meantime. Cook the pasta for 8 to 10 minutes, or until it is al dente, before draining it from the water.

Toss the hot pasta with the sauce and top with Parmesan cheese to finish it off!

Servings: 1 | Prep: 3 minutes, Cooking: 1h30 minutes, Total Time: 1h33 minutes BAKED POTATO | Prep: 3 minutes, Cooking: 1h30 minutes FACTS ABOUT VEGETABLE NUTRITION

One hundred twenty-eight calories | thirty-seven grams of carbohydrates | one hundred and twenty-seven grams of protein | zero milligrams of cholesterol

INGREDIENTS 1 baking potato (optional)

DIRECTIONS

350 degrees Fahrenheit for the oven (175 degrees C).

To prevent steam from building up and causing the potato to explode in your oven, scrub and prick it with a fork after it has been steamed.

1 1/2 hours in the oven

HOMEMADE BEANS IN A SLOW COOKER

| Prep time: 20 minutes | Cooking time: 10 minutes | Total time: 10 minutes and 20 seconds Nutritional Information: 296 calories | 57 grams of carbohydrate | 3 grams of fat | 12.4 grams of protein | 5 milligrams of cholesterol

INGREDIENTS

3 cups dried navy beans, soaked overnight or boiled for 1 hour.

mustard powder (about 1 tablespoon)

1 1/2 cups ketchup (or whatever you prefer)

Salt (one tablespoon)

water (approximately 1.5 cups)

6 slices thickly sliced bacon, cut into 1-inch chunks.

molasses (about 1/4 cup)

Brown sugar (about 1 cup)

chopped 1 medium-sized onion

DIRECTIONS

Remove the beans from the soaking liquid and place them in a Slow Cooker to cook on low for several hours.

Toss the beans in a large mixing bowl and stir in the ketchup, water, molasses, onion, mustard, salt, bacon, and brown sugar until everything is evenly distributed.

Cook on LOW for 8 to 10 hours, stirring occasionally if possible, but not necessary, for the best flavor.

WITH ROSEMARY AND BUTTERNUT SQUASH PIZZA

Approximately 50 minutes total time: 20 minutes for preparation, 30 minutes for cooking, and 20 minutes for total. Nutritional Information: 567 calories | 96.9 grams of carbohydrates | 13.7 grams of fat | 14.8 grams of protein | 3 milligrams of cholesterol

INGREDIENTS

34 cup of onion, thinly sliced

Divide the olive oil into three equal parts and set aside.

Half of a butternut squash, peeled, seeded, and thinly sliced

1 (16-ounce) package of refrigerated pizza crust dough, divided

freshly chopped rosemary (about 1 teaspoon)

To taste, add 1 tablespoon cornmeal, salt, and freshly ground black pepper.

Grated Asiago or Parmesan cheese (about 2 tablespoons)

DIRECTIONS

Bake at 400 degrees Fahrenheit for 20 minutes (205 degrees C). In a roasting pan, combine the sliced onion and squash. Using your hands, toss the vegetables in the rosemary, salt, and pepper, as well as 2 tablespoons of the olive oil.

Bake for 20 minutes, or until the onions are lightly browned and the squash is tender; remove from the oven and set aside.

Fahrenheit (450 degrees Fahrenheit) in the oven (230 degrees C). Roll out each ball of dough into an 8-inch round on a floured work surface. Prepare a baking sheet with cornmeal and arrange the rounds on it (you may need 2 baking sheets depending on their size). Make two rounds with the squash mixture and bake for another 10 minutes, checking on it every few minutes, or until the crust is set. Cheese and the remaining tablespoon of olive oil should be sprinkled on top before serving. Serve after cutting into quarters.

Chapter Five

BLACK BEANS AND RICE IN QUICK TIME

Prepare: 5 minutes; cook: 15 minutes; total preparation and preparation: 25 minutes. FACTS ABOUT VEGETABLE NUTRITION

Two hundred and seventy-one calories; 47.8g carbohydrate; 5.3g fat; 10g protein; and 0mg cholesterol

INGREDIENTS

1/4 cup lard or other cooking fat

dried oregano (1 teaspoon)

1-inch piece of onion, diced

garlic powder (1/2 teaspoon)

uncooked black beans from a 15-ounce can (without the water)

1 uncooked instant brown rice (about 1/2 cup).

Stew tomatoes (14.5 ounces) 1 (14.5 ounce) can

3. Pour in the oil and heat over medium heat until shimmering. Cook, stirring constantly, until the onion is soft. Combine the beans, tomatoes, oregano, and garlic powder in a large mixing bowl until well combined. Toss in the rice after the water has come to a boil. Stir occasionally for 5 minutes after covering with foil. After removing the pan from the heat, allow it to cool for 5 minutes before serving it.

DON'T WAIT TO MAKE THESE IN ADVANCE!

Prepare: 5 minutes; cook: 20 minutes; total preparation and preparation: 25 minutes. FACTS ABOUT VEGETABLE NUTRITION

363 calories | 46.1 grams of carbohydrate | 7.1 grams of fat | 28.1 grams of protein | 26 milligrams of cholesterol

INGREDIENTS

Macaroni and cheese mix (one package, 7.25 ounces)

Drain 1 can tuna (about 9 ounces) before using.

Condensed cream of mushroom soup (one can, or 10.75 ounces) 1

Peas (one ten-ounce can, drained):

DIRECTIONS 1. Prepare the macaroni and cheese mix according to the directions on the box. Combine the cream of mushroom soup, tuna, and peas in a large mixing bowl until thoroughly combined. Heat until bubbly, stirring frequently.

CHICKPEA AND SPINACH CUISINE

| Prep time: 5 minutes | Cooking time: 15 minutes |
Total time: 20 minutes 4 servings FACTS ABOUT VEGETABLE NUTRITION

346 calories | 44.7 grams of carbohydrate | 12.3 grams of fat | 21.7 grams of protein | 0 milligrams of cholesterol

INGREDIENTS

1/4 cup lard or other cooking fat

1/2 teaspoon garlic powder, or more to your personal preference

1-inch-thick slice of onion, finely chopped 1-can (15-ounce-size) garbanzo beans (chickpeas), drained and rinsed-off

1 can creamed corn (14.75 ounces)

firm tofu, cubed, 1 (12-ounce) package (1 tablespoon) curry paste

salt and pepper to taste 1 bunch fresh spinach (with stems removed)

to taste 1 teaspoon dried basil, or to taste 1 teaspoon freshly ground black pepper

DIRECTIONS

Sauté the onions until translucent in a large wok or skillet coated with oil over medium heat. Creamed corn and curry paste are added at the end of the cooking process. Stir frequently for 5 minutes, until the sauce has thickened. Season with salt, pepper, and garlic while stirring constantly.

In a separate bowl, combine garbanzo beans and tofu. Cover with the spinach. Remove the spinach from the heat and stir in the basil until it is fully incorporated into the dish.

SCAMPI SCAMPI SCAMPI SCAMPI SCAMPI SCAMPI SCAMPI SCAMPI

Approximately 45 minutes total time: 15 minutes for preparation, 30 minutes for cooking, and 15 minutes for cleaning FACTS ABOUT VEGETABLE NUTRITION

Nutritional Information (360 calories, 43.5 grams of carbohydrates, 9.3 grams of fat, 21.3 grams of protein, 31 mg of cholesterol)

INGREDIENTS

1 stick margarine (about 4 tablespoons)

3 garlic cloves, minced, 1/2 cup grated Romano cheese

1 chicken broth can (10.75 ounces) 1 large onion, minced

Bay scallops weighing 1 pound

white wine (dry) half a cup

Linguine pasta (about 1 pound)

Salt (about 1 teaspoon)

Fresh chopped parsley (about 1/4 cup)

peppercorns, 1/4 teaspoon freshly ground

DIRECTIONS

Garlic and onion should be sautéed until translucent in a large skillet melted with margarine over medium heat Using a fork, mash together 1/4 cup cheese, wine, salt, and freshly ground black pepper.

Increase the heat to high and bring the scallops to a rapid boil for 7 to 8 minutes, stirring constantly.

Prepare a large pot of lightly salted water to boil in the meantime. Cook the pasta for 8 to 10 minutes, or until it is al dente, before draining it from the water.

Remove pan from heat and stir in parsley; pour sauce over linguine and serve immediately. Lastly, top with the remaining cheese and serve immediately.

TOSSE PASTA IN TWELVE MINUTES.

16 minutes | 20 minutes preparation | 12 minutes cooking total time | 32 minutes preparation and cooking time. FACTS ABOUT VEGETABLE NUTRITION

360 calories | 46.3 grams of carbohydrate | 10.2 grams of fat | 21.4 grams of protein | 33 milligrams of cholesterol

INGREDIENTS

Rotini pasta (eighteen ounces), 1 1/4 teaspoon garlic powder, Olive oil (about 4 tblsp)

one-and-a-quarter teaspoon dried basil

cut into bite-size pieces four skinless, boneless chicken breast halves

dried oregano (1 1/4 teaspoons)

1 pound minced garlic (about 3 cloves)

1 cup sun-dried tomato pieces, finely chopped

salt (approximately 14 teaspoons)

grated cheese parmesan (about 1/4 cup)

DIRECTIONS

Boil the rotini in a large pot of lightly salted water for about 8 minutes, or until they are tender but still firm to the bite. Drain well.

Over medium-high heat, heat the oil in a large pot until shimmering. 5 to 10 minutes or until chicken is no longer pink in the middle, saute the chicken with the garlic, salt, garlic powder, basil, and oregano in hot oil. Cook for about 2 minutes, until the sun-dried tomatoes are heated through. Take the pan off the stovetop and put it somewhere safe to cool.

In a large mixing bowl, combine the pasta, chicken, and parmesan. Parmesan cheese should be sprinkled on top.

THE BURGERS MADE FROM GRILLED CHICKEN

Making 8 servings will take 30 minutes. Prepping will take 15 minutes. Cooking will take 15 minutes. FACTS ABOUT VEGETABLE NUTRITION

486 calories | 104 grams of carbohydrate | 4.7 grams of fat | 14.5 grams of protein | 23 milligrams of cholesterol

INGREDIENTS

1-inch piece of onion, diced

minced garlic 2 teaspoons ground chicken 2 lbs ground chicken

Egg (a single one).

half a cup fresh bread crumbs 1 red bell pepper, chopped

mushrooms, 1 cup, freshly sliced

old bay seasoning (to taste) 1 tbsp.

Toss 1 tomato with kosher salt to taste after it has been seeded.

2 carrots, chopped black pepper to taste, and 2 tablespoons olive oil

DIRECTIONS

Lightly oil the grate of an outdoor grill before turning it on medium heat.

Using a cooking or oil spray, lightly coat a saute pan over medium heat and place it on the stovetop. Stir-fry the onion and garlic first, then add the bell pepper and cook until soft. Add the mushrooms and tomatoes and cook until they are tender, stirring occasionally. Leave all of the vegetables to cool completely before storing them.

Toss the chicken and vegetables together in a large bowl. Season with salt and pepper to taste after adding the egg and bread crumbs. Prepare 8 patties by mixing everything together thoroughly.

Grill for 5 to 6 minutes per side, or until desired doneness is reached, over medium heat, turning halfway through.

CILANTRO SALMON GRILLED OVER HEAT

Cooking Time: 20 Minutes | Total Time: 45 Minutes | Servings: 6 FACTS ABOUT VEGETABLE NUTRITION

Four hundred fifty-nine calories, ninety-four grams of carbohydrates, four grams of fat, seventeen grams of protein, and thirty-four milligrams of cholesterol

INGREDIENTS

1 bunch cilantro leaves, finely chopped lime juice 1 lime (optional).

3-4 salmon steaks 2 garlic cloves, chopped

honey (to taste), 2 cups, salt and pepper

DIRECTIONS

In a small saucepan set over medium-low heat, combine the cilantro, garlic, honey, and lime juice until the cilantro is tender. Continue to cook for about 5 minutes, or until the honey can be stirred easily. Remove the pan from the heat and set it aside to cool for a few moments.

Season the salmon steaks with salt and pepper in a baking dish before baking. Refrigerate for 10 minutes after pouring marinade over salmon.

Set a high heat setting on an outdoor grill to prepare it for use.

Grease the grill grate with a light coating of cooking spray. Salmon steaks should be cooked for 5 minutes on each side, or until the fish can be flaked easily with a fork, should be placed on the grill.

STIR-FRY OF JAPANESE BEEF

Making 8 servings will take 30 minutes. Prepping will take 15 minutes. Cooking will take 15 minutes. FACTS ABOUT VEGETABLE NUTRITION

290 calories | 26.4 grams of carbohydrate | 7.6 grams of fat | 26.4 grams of protein | 39 milligrams of cholesterol

INGREDIENTS

Boneless beef sirloin or beef top round steaks (approximately 3/4 inch thick): 2 lbs.

2 lbs shiitake mushrooms, thinly sliced

1 cup cornstarch (about 3 tablespoons)

Chinese cabbage (bok choy) 1 (10.5 ounce) can Campbell's Condensed Beef Broth 1 (10.5 ounce) can Campbell's Condensed Chicken Broth

3 large peppers (medium size), cut into 2-inch-long strips

Soy sauce (1/2 cup)

celery, sliced into thirds 3 celery stalks 2 tablespoons sugar

cut 2 medium green onions into 2" pieces 2 medium green onions

vegetable oil (around 2 tbsp.)

Long-grain white rice that has been heated to a boil

DIRECTIONS

Very thin strips of beef should be used.

Combine the cornstarch, broth, soy sauce, and sugar in a large mixing bowl until smooth and well combined. Make a note of it.

In a saucepot or wok, heat 1 tablespoon of oil over high heat until shimmering and fragrant. Stir-fry the beef in two batches until it is browned on each side. Make a separate place for the beef.

1 tbsp. extra virgin olive oil Using two batches, stir-fry the vegetables until they are tender-crisp but not mushy over

medium heat until the mushrooms are softened. Make a place for the vegetables.

Add the cornstarch mixture after it has been thoroughly stirred together. Keep stirring constantly until the mixture comes to a boil and thickens. Cook until the beef and vegetables are thoroughly heated. Toss with rice and enjoy!

GREEN BEANS WITH A CRACKER

Prepare for four servings in ten minutes, cook for twenty minutes, then cook for the whole thirty minutes. FACTS ABOUT VEGETABLE NUTRITION

101 calories | 16.4 grams of carbohydrate | 3.7 grams of fat | 4.2 grams of protein | 0 milligrams of cholesterol

INGREDIENTS

Fresh green beans, trimmed (about 2 pounds)

1 teaspoon fine sea salt (kosher)

or as needed, 1 tablespoon extra-virgin olive oil

peppercorns that have been freshly ground

DIRECTIONS

Bake at 400 degrees Fahrenheit for 20 minutes (200 degrees C).

If necessary, pat the green beans dry with paper towels before spreading them out on a jellyroll pan to cool completely. Season with salt and pepper after drizzling with olive oil. Spread the beans out so they don't overlap and coat them evenly with olive oil with your fingers.

Roast the beans in the preheated oven for 20 to 25 minutes, or until they are slightly shriveled and spotted with brown spots.

RICE WITH EGGS IN IT

| Prep time: 5 minutes | Cooking time: 15 minutes | Total time: 20 minutes 4 servings FACTS ABOUT VEGETABLE NUTRITION

145 calories | 24.6 grams of carbohydrate | 2.7 grams of fat | 4.9 grams of protein | 46 milligrams of cholesterol

INGREDIENTS

Water (one cup)

finely chopped half an onion

salt (half a teaspoon)

green beans (about half a cup).

soy sauce (about 2 tablespoons)

1 lightly beaten egg (optional).

instant white rice (uncooked) 1 cup

peppercorns, 1/4 teaspoon freshly ground

vegetable oil (about 1 tbsp.)

DIRECTIONS

Boil the water with the salt and soy sauce in a saucepan until the water is clear. Stir in the rice until it is well-combined. After removing the pan from the heat, cover it and set it aside for five minutes.

Over medium heat, heat the oil in a medium skillet or wok. For 2 to 3 minutes, sauté the onions and green beans. In a separate pan, heat the oil over medium heat for 2 minutes, scrambling the egg as it cooks.

In a large mixing bowl, combine the cooked rice, salt, and pepper; mix well.

PASTA WITH BROCCOLI AND CHICKEN

| Prep time: 10 minutes | Cooking time: 10 minutes | Total time: 20 minutes | 8 servings FACTS ABOUT VEGETABLE NUTRITION

368 calories | 51 grams of carbohydrate | 7.7 grams of fat | 23.5 grams of protein | 34 milligrams of cholesterol

INGREDIENTS

Salt and pepper to taste with 3 tablespoons extra-virgin olive oil

chicken breast halves (1 pound, skinless, boneless) - cut into 1-inch pieces

dried oregano (about a teaspoonful)

chopped onion (about 1 tablespoon total)

penne pasta (dried, 18 oz.)

2 garlic cloves, peeled and minced

1/4 cup thinly sliced fresh basil leaves (optional)

tomato sauce (from 2 (14.5 ounce) cans)

2 tbsp. grated Parmesan cheese (optional).

Fresh broccoli florets (about 2 cups)

DIRECTIONS

Over medium heat, warm the oil in a large skillet before adding the chicken and cooking until it is slightly browned.

Cook for 5 minutes, or until the garlic is golden and the onions are translucent, after which remove from heat.

Season with salt and pepper and stir in the oregano before bringing the pot to a boil over high heat. For approximately 10 minutes, cover and reduce the heat to a simmer.

Prepare a large pot of lightly salted water to boil in the meantime. Cook for 8 to 10 minutes, or until the pasta is tender, then drain and return to the pot. In a large mixing bowl, combine chicken sauce and water.

Sprinkle with Parmesan cheese after adding the basil. Serve.

A QUINOA WITH LEMONY

Cooking Time: 10 Minutes | Total Time: 25 Minutes | Servings: 6 FACTS ABOUT VEGETABLE NUTRITION

147 calories | 21.4 grams of carbohydrate | 4.8 grams of fat | 5.9 grams of protein | 0 milligrams of cholesterol

INGREDIENTS

Chop 2 celery stalks and 1/4 cup pine nuts.

quinoa (one cup)

water and a quarter of a red onion, chopped

cayenne pepper (to taste) 1/4 teaspoon sea salt

ground cumin (half a teaspoon)

fresh lemon juice (about a quarter cup)

2 tablespoons finely chopped fresh parsley

DIRECTIONS

In a dry skillet over medium heat, toast the pine nuts until fragrant. The cooking time will be approximately 5 minutes, with constant stirring because they will easily burn. Leave to cool for a moment.

Cooking instructions: Combine the quinoa, water, and salt in a saucepan over medium heat. After bringing the water to a boil, reduce heat to medium and continue to cook until the quinoa is tender and the water has been completely absorbed, approximately 10 minutes. Allow to cool for a few minutes before fluffing with a spatula.

Add in the pine nuts, lemon juice, celery, onion, cayenne pepper, cumin, and parsley to the quinoa in a large mixing bowl and toss to combine. Before serving, taste and adjust the seasonings if necessary.

VEGETABLE SAUCE WITH FROZEN INGREDIENTS.

| Prep time: 5 minutes, Cook time: 5 minutes, Total preparation time: 10 minutes. FACTS ABOUT VEGETABLE NUTRITION

This recipe contains 88 calories, 13.8 grams of carbohydrates, 2.9 grams of fat, 3.5 grams of protein, and zero milligrams of cholesterol.

INGREDIENTS

soy sauce (about 2 tablespoons)

2 teaspoons peanut butter (or other nut butter of choice).

Brown sugar (one tablespoon)

oil (olive) (two teaspoons)

Garlic powder (two teaspoons)

Frozen mixed vegetables, one (16-ounce) package

DIRECTIONS

In a small bowl, whisk together the soy sauce, brown sugar, garlic powder, and peanut butter.

Cook and stir frozen vegetables until they are just tender, 5 to 7 minutes, in a large skillet coated with oil over medium heat. Stir in soy sauce mixture after removing the pan from the heat

BALSAMIC CHICKEN COOKED ON THE SLOW STOVE

| Prep 15 minutes | Cooking Time 4 hours and 15 minutes | Total Time: 4 hours and 15 minutes FACTS ABOUT VEGETABLE NUTRITION

Amount per serving: 200 calories | 17.6 grams of carbohydrates | 6.8 grams of fat | 18.6 grams of protein | 43 milligrams of cholesterol

INGREDIENTS

olive oil (around 2 tbsp.

1 tbsp. dry basil, chopped

1 pound chicken breast halves, skinless and boneless (or more to your liking).

1/4 cup finely ground black pepper and 1 teaspoon dried rosemary salt (to taste)

1/2 teaspoon thyme leaves, dried

onion, thinly sliced (approximately 1)

1/2 cup balsamic vinegar

4 cloves garlic

2 (14.5 ounce) cans crushed tomatoes

dried oregano (1 teaspoon)

DIRECTIONS

Drizzle olive oil into the slow cooker. Place chicken breasts on top of oil and season each breast with salt and pepper. Top chicken breasts with onion slices, garlic, oregano, basil, rosemary, and thyme. Drizzle balsamic vinegar over seasoned breasts and pour tomatoes on top.

Cook in the slow cooker set to High until chicken is no longer pink in the center and the juices run clear, about 4 hours.

ZUCCHINI COOKIES

Servings: 36 | Prep: 15m | Cooks: 10m | Total: 25m

NUTRITION FACTS\sCalories: 81 | Carbohydrates: 13.4g | Fat: 2.7g | Protein: 1g | Cholesterol: 5mg

INGREDIENTS

1/2 cup margarine, softened

1 teaspoon baking soda

1 cup white sugar

1/2 teaspoon salt\s1 egg

1 teaspoon ground cinnamon

1 cup grated zucchini

1/2 teaspoon ground cloves

2 cups all-purpose flour

1 cup raisins

DIRECTIONS

In a medium bowl, cream together the margarine and sugar until smooth. Beat in the egg then stir in the zucchini. Combine the flour, baking soda, salt and cinnamon; stir into the zucchini mixture. Mix in raisins. Cover dough and chill for at least 1 hour or overnight.

Oven should be preheated at 375 degrees Fahrenheit (190 degrees C). Grease cookie sheets. Drop dough by teaspoonfuls onto the prepared cookie sheet. Cookies should be about 2 inches apart.

Bake for 8 to 10 minutes in the preheated oven until set. Allow cookies to cool slightly on the cookie sheets before removing to wire racks to cool completely.

MY FAVORITE SESAME NOODLES

Servings: 1 | Prep: 10m | Cooks: 15m | Total: 25m FACTS ABOUT VEGETABLE NUTRITION

Calories: 787 | Carbohydrates: 114.6g | Fat: 26.1g | Protein: 28.3g | Cholesterol: 0mg

INGREDIENTS

1/2 (8 ounce) package spaghetti

1 teaspoon sesame oil 2 tablespoons peanut butter ground ginger (one teaspoon)

1 tablespoon honey 1 clove garlic, minced

2 tablespoons tamari

1 green onion, peeled and finely minced

1 teaspoon Thai chili sauce

2 teaspoons sesame seeds

DIRECTIONS

Fill a large pot with lightly salted water and bring to a rolling boil over high heat. Once the water is boiling, stir in the spaghetti, and return to a boil. Cook the pasta uncovered, stirring occasionally, until the pasta has cooked through, but is still firm to the bite, about 12 minutes. Drain well in a colander set in the sink.

Melt the peanut butter in a large microwave-safe glass or ceramic bowl, 15 to 20 seconds (depending on your microwave). Whisk the honey, tamari, and chili sauce into the peanut butter, then stir in the sesame oil and ginger. Mix in the garlic and green onions and toss with the spaghetti. Top with the sesame seeds.

GARLIC CHICKEN FRIED BROWN RICE

Servings: 3 | Prep: 20m | Cooks: 15m | Total: 35m FACTS ABOUT VEGETABLE NUTRITION

Calories: 444 | Carbohydrates: 57.4g | Fat: 12.8g | Protein: 24.3g | Cholesterol: 43mg

INGREDIENTS

2 tablespoons vegetable oil, divided 3 cups cooked brown rice

8 ounces skinless, boneless chicken breast, cut into strips

2 tablespoons light soy sauce

1/2 red bell pepper, chopped 1 tablespoon rice vinegar

1/2 cup green onion, chopped 1 cup frozen peas, thawed 4 cloves garlic, minced

DIRECTIONS

Heat 1 tablespoon of vegetable oil in a large skillet set over medium heat. Add the chicken, bell pepper, green onion and garlic. Cook and stir until the chicken is cooked through, about 5 minutes. Remove the chicken to a plate and keep warm.

Heat the remaining tablespoon of oil in the same skillet over medium-high heat. Add the rice; cook and stir to heat through. Stir in the soy sauce, rice vinegar and peas, and continue to cook for 1 minute. Return the chicken mixture to the skillet and stir to blend with the rice and heat through before serving.

EASY MASOOR DAAL

Prepare: 5 minutes; cook: 30 minutes; total preparation and cooking time: 35 minutes. FACTS ABOUT VEGETABLE NUTRITION

Calories: 185 | Carbohydrates: 25g | Fat: 5.2g | Protein: 11.1g | Cholesterol: 0mg

INGREDIENTS

1 cup red lentils

1/2 teaspoon cayenne pepper, or to taste

1 slice ginger, 1 inch piece, peeled

4 teaspoons vegetable oil

1/4 teaspoon ground turmeric

4 teaspoons dried minced onion 1 teaspoon salt 1 teaspoon cumin seeds

DIRECTIONS

Rinse lentils thoroughly and place in a medium saucepan along with ginger, turmeric, salt and cayenne pepper. Cover with about 1 inch of water and bring to a boil. Skim off any foam that forms on top of the lentils. Reduce heat and simmer, stirring occasionally, until beans are tender and soupy.

Meanwhile, in a microwave safe dish combine oil, dried onion and cumin seeds. Microwave on high for 45 seconds to 1 minute; be sure to brown, but not burn, onions. Stir into lentil mixture.

MEXICAN RICE

Servings: 7 | Prep: 15m | Cooks: 30m | Total: 45m FACTS ABOUT VEGETABLE NUTRITION

Calories: 79 | Carbohydrates: 15.1g | Fat: 1.2g | Protein: 1.5g | Cholesterol: 0mg

INGREDIENTS

1 1/2 teaspoons vegetable oil

1/2 teaspoon chili powder

1/2 small small onion, diced 3 ounces canned diced tomatoes

2/3 cup uncooked long-grain rice

Salt (about 1 teaspoon)

ground cumin (half a teaspoon)

water (approximately 1.5 cups)

DIRECTIONS

In a large saucepan, heat oil over medium heat. Stir in onion and saute until translucent.

Pour the rice into the pan and stir to coat grains with oil. Mix in cumin, chili powder, tomatoes, salt and water. Cover, bring to a boil then reduce heat to low. Cook at a simmer for 20 to 30 minutes or until rice is tender. Stir occasionally.

BAKED SCALLOPED POTATOES

Servings: 8 | Prep: 15m | Cooks: 1h15m | Total: 1h30m FACTS ABOUT VEGETABLE NUTRITION

Calories: 234 | Carbohydrates: 41g | Fat: 3.3g | Protein: 9g | Cholesterol: 3mg

INGREDIENTS

6 large peeled, cubed potatoes

1 onion, diced 1 (10.75 ounce) can condensed cream of mushroom soup

peppercorns, 1/2 teaspoon freshly ground

1 1/4 cups milk

DIRECTIONS

Oven should be preheated at 375 degrees Fahrenheit (190 degrees C). Grease a 2 quart casserole dish.

Layer potatoes and onions into the casserole dish. Combine soup, milk and pepper in a bowl, then pour soup mixture over the potatoes and onions. The soup mixture should almost cover the potatoes and onion, if it does not add extra milk.

Cover dish and bake in preheated 375 degrees F (190 degrees C) oven for 60 minutes or until the potatoes are cooked through. At 30 minutes, remove the casserole from the oven and stir once before returning the dish to the oven. Remove from oven and serve.

GOBI ALOO (INDIAN STYLE CAULIFLOWER WITH POTATOES)

Approximately 35 minutes total time: 15 minutes for preparation, 20 minutes for cooking. FACTS ABOUT VEGETABLE NUTRITION

Calories: 135 | Carbohydrates: 23.1g | Fat: 4g | Protein: 4g | Cholesterol: 0mg

INGREDIENTS

1/4 cup lard or other cooking fat

1/2 teaspoon paprika

1 teaspoon cumin seeds

1 teaspoon cumin seeds (ground)

1 teaspoon minced garlic, preferably fresh.

1/2 teaspoon garam masala

1 teaspoon ginger paste

depending on your own preference

2 medium potatoes, peeled and cubed

1 pound cauliflower

1/2 teaspoon ground turmeric

1 teaspoon chopped fresh cilantro

DIRECTIONS

Heat the oil in a medium skillet over medium heat. Stir in the cumin seeds, garlic, and ginger paste. Cook about 1 minute until garlic is lightly browned. Add the potatoes. Season with turmeric, paprika, cumin, garam masala, and salt. Cover and continue cooking 5 to 7 minutes stirring occasionally.

Mix the cauliflower and cilantro into the saucepan. Reduce heat to low and cover. Stirring occasionally, continue cooking 10 minutes, or until potatoes and cauliflower are tender.

KIKI'S BORRACHO (DRUNKEN) BEANS Servings: 12 | Prep: 30m | Cooks: 3h | Total: 3h30m FACTS ABOUT VEGETABLE NUTRITION

Calories: 181 | Carbohydrates: 31.8g | Fat: 1g | Protein: 9.6g | Cholesterol: 0mg

INGREDIENTS

1 pound dried pinto beans, washed

1 white onion, diced

2 quarts chicken stock

1/4 cup pickled jalapeno peppers

1 tablespoon salt 6 cloves garlic, chopped

1/2 tablespoon ground black pepper

3 bay leaves

1 (12 fluid ounce) can or bottle dark beer

1 1/2 tablespoons dried oregano

2 (14.5 ounce) cans chopped stewed tomatoes

1 1/2 cups chopped fresh cilantro

DIRECTIONS

Soak beans in a large pot of water overnight.

Drain beans, and refill the pot with chicken stock and enough water to cover the beans with 2 inches of liquid. Sea salt and freshly ground pepper are added for seasoning. Cover, and bring to a boil. Reduce heat to medium- low, cover, and cook for 1 1/2 hours. Stir the beans occasionally through out the entire cooking process to make sure they do not burn or stick to the bottom of the pot.

Stir beer, tomatoes, onion, jalapeno peppers, garlic, bay leaves, oregano, and cilantro into the beans. Continue to cook uncovered for 1 hour, or until beans are tender.

With a potato masher, crush the beans slightly to thicken the bean liquid. Adjust the seasonings with salt and pepper to taste.

CUBAN BEANS AND RICE

Servings: 6 | Prep: 10m | Cooks: 50m | Total: 1h NUTRITION FACTS

Calories: 258 | Carbohydrates: 49.3g | Fat: 3.2g | Protein: 7.3g | Cholesterol: 2mg

INGREDIENTS

olive oil (around 1 tablespoon)

1 teaspoon salt 1 cup chopped onion 4 tablespoons tomato paste

1 green bell pepper, chopped 1 (15.25 ounce) can kidney beans, drained with liquid reserved

garlic, minced (about 2 cloves total)

1 cup uncooked white rice

DIRECTIONS

Heat oil in a large saucepan over medium heat. Saute onion, bell pepper and garlic. When onion is translucent add salt and tomato paste. Reduce heat to low and cook 2 minutes. Stir in the beans and rice.

Pour the liquid from the beans into a large measuring cup and add enough water to reach a volume of 2 1/2 cups; pour into beans. Cover and cook on low for 45 to 50 minutes, or until liquid is absorbed and rice is cooked.

CILANTRO-LIME RICE

Servings: 6 | Prep: 5m | Cooks: 25m | Total: 30m FACTS ABOUT VEGETABLE NUTRITION

Calories: 115 | Carbohydrates: 25.2g | Fat: 0.g | Protein: 2.3g | Cholesterol: 1mg

INGREDIENTS

1 cup long grain white rice

2 tbsp. lime juice (from fresh)

2 cups water 2 tablespoons chopped fresh cilantro

1 teaspoon chicken bouillon granules

depending on your own preference

DIRECTIONS 1. Bring the rice, water, and chicken bouillon to a boil in a saucepan over high heat. Reduce heat to medium-low, cover, and simmer until the rice is tender, 20 to 25 minutes. Remove from the heat, add the lime juice, cilantro, and salt; fluff with a fork and serve.

3. Heat the olive oil in a saucepan over low heat; add the green beans to the hot oil and cover the saucepan. Pour the

green beans and sauce into the pan and cook, shaking the pan regularly, until the beans are slightly tender, about 5 minutes.

HEALTHIER OVEN ROASTED POTATOES

Approximately 35 minutes total time: 15 minutes for preparation, 20 minutes for cooking. NUTRITION FACTS Calories: 319 | Carbohydrates: 65.5g | Fat: 3.8g | Protein: 7.7g | Cholesterol: 0mg

INGREDIENTS

olive oil (around 1 tablespoon)

Fresh chopped parsley (about 1 teaspoon)

1 tablespoon minced garlic, preferably fresh.

1/2 teaspoon red pepper flakes

freshly chopped basil (about 1 tablespoon total)

salt (half a teaspoon)

1 tablespoon chopped fresh rosemary

Peeled and diced potatoes (four big potatoes)

DIRECTIONS

400 degrees Fahrenheit for the oven (245 degrees C).

Combine oil, garlic, basil, rosemary, parsley, red pepper flakes, and salt in a large bowl. Toss in potatoes until evenly coated. Using a roasting pan or baking sheet, arrange the potatoes in a single layer.

Roast in preheated oven, turning occasionally, until potatoes are brown on all sides, 20 to 30 minutes.

EX-GIRLFRIEND'S MOM'S SALSA FRESCA (PICO DE GALLO)

Servings: 6 | Prep: 20m | Cooks: 20m | Total: 40m | Additional: 20m FACTS ABOUT VEGETABLE NUTRITION

Calories: 29 | Carbohydrates: 6.9g | Fat: 0.2g | Protein: 1.1g | Cholesterol: 0mg

INGREDIENTS

1 cup finely chopped red onion

2 1/2 cups Roma (plum) tomatoes, seeded and chopped

1 jalapeno pepper, seeded and finely chopped - or more to taste

1/2 cup chopped fresh cilantro

2 limes, juiced 1 teaspoon salt

DIRECTIONS 1. Mix red onion, jalapeno pepper, and lime juice in a bowl. Allow to stand for 5 minutes. Mix in Roma tomatoes, cilantro, and salt; allow to stand 15 more minutes for flavors to blend.

BLACK BEAN SALSA

Servings: 40 | Prep: 15m | Cooks: 8h | Total: 8h15m | Additional: 8h NUTRITION FACTS Calories: 42 | Carbohydrates: 8.3g | Fat: 0.2g | Protein: 2.5g | Cholesterol: 0mg

INGREDIENTS

3 (15 ounce) cans black beans, drained and rinsed 2 tomatoes, diced 1 (11 ounce) can Mexican-style corn, drained 2 bunches green onions, chopped 2 (10 ounce) cans diced tomatoes with green chile peppers, partially drained cilantro leaves, for garnish

DIRECTIONS 1. In a large bowl, mix together black beans, Mexican-style corn, diced tomatoes with green chile peppers, tomatoes and green onion stalks. Garnish with desired amount of cilantro leaves. Chill in the refrigerator at least 8 hours, or overnight, before serving.

Chapter Seven

THAI SPICY BASIL CHICKEN FRIED RICE

Servings: 6 | Prep: 30m | Cooks: 10m | Total: 40m NUTRITION FACTS Calories: 794 | Carbohydrates: 116.4g | Fat: 22.1g | Protein: 29.1g | Cholesterol: 46mg

INGREDIENTS

3 tablespoons oyster sauce

1 pound boneless, skinless chicken breast, cut into thin strips

2 tablespoons fish sauce

1 red pepper, seeded and thinly sliced

sugar (white) - 1 teaspoon

onion, thinly sliced (approximately 1)

1/2 cup peanut oil for frying

2 cups sweet Thai basil

4 cups cooked jasmine rice, chilled

1 cucumber, sliced (optional)

6 large cloves garlic clove, crushed

1/2 cup cilantro sprigs (optional)

2 serrano peppers, crushed

DIRECTIONS

Whisk together the oyster sauce, fish sauce, and sugar in a bowl.

Heat the oil in a wok over medium-high heat until the oil begins to smoke. Add the garlic and serrano peppers, stirring quickly. Stir in the chicken, bell pepper, onion and oyster sauce mixture; cook until the chicken is no longer pink. Raise heat to high and stir in the chilled rice; stir quickly until the sauce is blended with the rice. Use the back of a spoon to break up any rice sticking together.

Remove from heat and mix in the basil leaves. Garnish with sliced cucumber and cilantro as desired.

CAVATELLI AND BROCCOLI

Servings: 12 | Prep: 10m | Cooks: 25m | Total: 35m FACTS ABOUT VEGETABLE NUTRITION

Calories: 317 | Carbohydrates: 47.6g | Fat: 10.3g | Protein: 10.2g | Cholesterol: 1mg

INGREDIENTS

3 heads fresh broccoli, cut into florets

1 teaspoon salt 1/2 cup olive oil

1-teaspoon red pepper flakes that have been crushed

1 pound minced garlic (about 3 cloves)

2 tbsp. grated Parmesan cheese (optional).

DOREEN'S HAM SLICES ON THE GRILL

Servings: 4 | Prep: 10m | Cooks: 15m | Total: 25m FACTS ABOUT VEGETABLE NUTRITION

Calories: 245 | Carbohydrates: 58g | Fat: 1.3g | Protein: 2.7g | Cholesterol: 8mg

INGREDIENTS

1 cup packed brown sugar

1/3 cup prepared horseradish 1/4 cup lemon juice

2 slices ham

DIRECTIONS

Preheat an outdoor grill for high heat and lightly oil grate.

In a small bowl, mix brown sugar, lemon juice and prepared horseradish.

Heat the brown sugar mixture in the microwave on high heat 1 minute, or until warm.

Score both sides of ham slices. Place on the prepared grill. Baste continuously with the brown sugar mixture while grilling. Grill 6 to 8 minutes per side, or to desired doneness.

BROKEN SPAGHETTI RISOTTO

Servings: 2 | Prep: 10m | Cooks: 15m | Total: 25m FACTS ABOUT VEGETABLE NUTRITION

Calories: 518 | Carbohydrates: 86.3g | Fat: 10.5g | Protein: 17.8g | Cholesterol: 9mg

INGREDIENTS

olive oil (around 1 tablespoon)

1/2 teaspoon red pepper flakes, or to taste

8 ounces uncooked spaghetti, broken into 1 inch pieces salt to taste

garlic, minced (about 2 cloves total)

2 tablespoons freshly grated Parmigiano-Reggiano cheese, or to taste

1 1/2 cups chicken broth

1 tablespoon chopped fresh flat-leaf parsley

DIRECTIONS

Heat oil in a saucepan over medium heat; add spaghetti and toast, stirring constantly, until golden brown, 3 to 5 minutes.

Stir garlic into spaghetti pieces and cook for 30 seconds.

Pour in 1/2 cup broth and increase heat to medium high. Stir spaghetti and broth until all the liquid is absorbed, 2 to 3 minutes. Repeat this process until all of the stock is absorbed and noodles are desired tenderness, about 10 minutes.

Reduce heat to low. Season spaghetti with salt and red pepper flakes to taste. Take the pan off the stovetop and put it somewhere safe to cool.

Stir Parmigiano-Reggiano cheese and parsley into spaghetti and serve.

EASY LIMA BEANS

Servings: 6 | Prep: 15m | Cooks: 30m | Total: 45m FACTS ABOUT VEGETABLE NUTRITION

Calories: 84 | Carbohydrates: 15.9g | Fat: 0g | Protein: 4.1g | Cholesterol: 0mg

INGREDIENTS

cooking spray

1 1/2 cups chicken broth 1/2 medium onion, finely chopped

1 (16 ounce) package frozen baby lima beans

DIRECTIONS 1. Heat a large saucepan over medium heat, and spray with cooking spray. Saute onions until soft and translucent. Pour in chicken broth, and bring to a boil. Add lima beans, and enough water just to cover. Bring to a boil, then reduce heat to low, cover, and simmer for 30 minutes, until beans are tender.

CHICKEN YAKISOBA

Servings: 4 | Prep: 20m | Cooks: 15m | Total: 35m FACTS ABOUT VEGETABLE NUTRITION

Calories: 503 | Carbohydrates: 69.8g | Fat: 16.5g | Protein: 26.5g | Cholesterol: 29mg

INGREDIENTS

2 tablespoons canola oil

1/2 medium head cabbage, thinly sliced

1 tablespoon sesame oil

1 onion, sliced

cut 2 skinless, boneless chicken breast halves into bite-size pieces each

2 carrots, cut into matchsticks

garlic, minced (about 2 cloves total)

Salt (one tablespoon)

2 tablespoons Asian-style chile paste

2 pounds cooked yakisoba noodles

Soy sauce (1/2 cup)

2 tablespoons pickled ginger, or to taste (optional)

canola oil (about 1 tbsp.

DIRECTIONS

Heat 2 tablespoons canola oil and sesame oil in a large skillet over medium-high heat. Cook and stir chicken and garlic in hot oil until fragrant, about 1 minute. Stir chile paste into chicken mixture; cook and stir until chicken is completely browned, 3 to 4 minutes. Add soy sauce and simmer for 2 minutes. Pour chicken and sauce into a bowl.

Heat 1 tablespoon canola oil in the skillet over medium-high heat; cook and stir cabbage, onion, carrots, and salt in hot oil until cabbage is wilted, 3 to 4 minutes.

Stir the chicken mixture into the cabbage mixture. Add noodles; cook and stir until noodles are hot and chicken is no longer pink inside, 3 to 4 minutes. Garnish with pickled ginger.

ZUCCHINI WITH CHICKPEA AND MUSHROOM STUFFING

Servings: 8 | Prep: 30m | Cooks: 30m | Total: 1h NUTRITION FACTS Calories: 107 | Carbohydrates: 18.4g | Fat: 2.7g | Protein: 4.5g | Cholesterol: 0mg

INGREDIENTS

4 zucchini, halved 1 1/2 teaspoons ground cumin, or to taste olive oil (around 1 tablespoon)

1 (15.5 ounce) can chickpeas, rinsed and drained

1 onion, chopped 1/2 lemon, juiced 2 cloves garlic, crushed

2 tablespoons chopped fresh parsley

1/2 (8 ounce) package button mushrooms, sliced sea salt to taste

1 teaspoon ground coriander ground black pepper to taste

DIRECTIONS

350 degrees Fahrenheit for the oven (175 degrees C). Grease a shallow baking dish.

Scoop out the flesh of the zucchini; chop the flesh and set aside. Place the shells in the prepared dish.

Heat oil in a large skillet over medium heat. Saute onions for 5 minutes, then add garlic and saute 2 minutes more. Stir in chopped zucchini and mushrooms; saute 5 minutes. Stir in coriander, cumin, chickpeas, lemon juice, parsley, salt and pepper. Spoon mixture into zucchini shells.

Bake in preheated oven for 30 to 40 minutes, or until zucchini are tender.

SPINACH, RED LENTIL, AND BEAN CURRY

Servings: 4 | Prep: 25m | Cooks: 10m | Total: 35m NUTRITION FACTS Calories: 328 | Carbohydrates: 51.9g | Fat: 8.3g | Protein: 18g | Cholesterol: 2mg

INGREDIENTS

1 cup red lentils

1-inch piece of onion, diced

1/4 cup tomato puree

2 garlic cloves, peeled and minced

1/2 (8 ounce) container plain yogurt

1 (1 inch) piece fresh ginger root, grated

1 teaspoon garam masala

4 cups loosely packed fresh spinach, coarsely chopped

1/2 teaspoon ground dried turmeric

2 tomatoes, chopped

ground cumin (half a teaspoon)

4 sprigs fresh cilantro, chopped

1/2 teaspoon ancho chile powder

1 (15.5 ounce) can mixed beans, rinsed and drained

vegetable oil (around 2 tbsp.)

DIRECTIONS

Rinse lentils and place in a saucepan with enough water to cover. To bring to a boil, put the water in a saucepan. Reduce heat to low, cover pot, and simmer over low heat for 20 minutes. Drain.

In a bowl, stir together tomato puree and yogurt. Season with garam masala, turmeric, cumin, and chile powder. Stir until creamy.

Heat oil in a skillet over medium heat. Stir in onion, garlic, and ginger; cook until onion begins to brown. Stir in spinach; cook until dark green and wilted. Gradually stir in yogurt mixture. Then mix in tomatoes and cilantro.

Stir lentils and mixed beans into mixture until well combined. Heat through, about 5 minutes.

QUICK SESAME GREEN BEANS

Approximately 15 minutes total: 10 minutes for preparation, 5 minutes for cooking. FACTS ABOUT VEGETABLE NUTRITION

Calories: 45 | Carbohydrates: 7.1g | Fat: 1.4g | Protein: 2.3g | Cholesterol: 0mg

INGREDIENTS

8 ounces fresh green beans, trimmed

garlic, minced (four cloves)

2 tablespoons low sodium soy sauce

1 teaspoon grated fresh ginger root 1/2 tablespoon miso paste

1 tablespoon sesame seeds, toasted

1/2 teaspoon red pepper flakes

DIRECTIONS

Place the green beans into a steamer insert and set in a pot over one inch of water. Bring to a boil, cover and steam for 5 minutes. Remove from the heat and transfer beans to a serving bowl.

Meanwhile, in a small bowl, stir together the soy sauce, miso paste, red pepper flakes, garlic and ginger. Pour over the green beans and toss to coat. Sprinkle sesame seeds on top.

EMILY'S FAMOUS MARSHMALLOWS

Servings: 18 | Prep: 30m | Cooks: 20m | Total: 8h40m FACTS ABOUT VEGETABLE NUTRITION

Calories: 118 | Carbohydrates: 29.8g | Fat: 0g | Protein: 0.4g | Cholesterol: 0mg

INGREDIENTS

1 cup confectioners' sugar for dusting

4 tablespoons unflavored gelatin

2 cups white sugar 2 egg whites

1 tablespoon light corn syrup

1 teaspoon vanilla extract

1 1/4 cups water, divided

DIRECTIONS

Dust a 9x9 inch square dish generously with confectioners' sugar.

In a small saucepan over medium-high heat, stir together white sugar, corn syrup and 3/4 cup water. Heat to 250 to 265 degrees F (121 to 129 degrees C), or until a small amount of syrup dropped into cold water forms a rigid ball. • While syrup is heating, place remaining water in a metal bowl and sprinkle gelatin over the surface. Place bowl over simmering water until gelatin has dissolved completely. Keep in a warm place until syrup has come to temperature. Remove syrup from heat and whisk gelatin mixture into hot syrup. Make a note of it.

In a separate bowl, whip egg whites to soft peaks. Continue to beat, pouring syrup mixture into egg whites in a thin stream, until the egg whites are very stiff. Stir in vanilla. Spread evenly in prepared pan and let rest 8 hours or overnight before cutting.CAVATELLI AND BROCCOLI

Servings: 12 | Prep: 10m | Cooks: 25m | Total: 35m FACTS ABOUT VEGETABLE NUTRITION

Calories: 317 | Carbohydrates: 47.6g | Fat: 10.3g | Protein: 10.2g | Cholesterol: 1mg

INGREDIENTS

3 heads fresh broccoli, cut into florets

1 teaspoon salt 1/2 cup olive oil

1-teaspoon red pepper flakes that have been crushed

1 pound minced garlic (about 3 cloves)

2 tbsp. grated Parmesan cheese (optional).

DOREEN'S HAM SLICES ON THE GRILL

Servings: 4 | Prep: 10m | Cooks: 15m | Total: 25m FACTS ABOUT VEGETABLE NUTRITION

Calories: 245 | Carbohydrates: 58g | Fat: 1.3g | Protein: 2.7g | Cholesterol: 8mg

INGREDIENTS

1 cup packed brown sugar

1/3 cup prepared horseradish 1/4 cup lemon juice

2 slices ham

DIRECTIONS

Preheat an outdoor grill for high heat and lightly oil grate.

In a small bowl, mix brown sugar, lemon juice and prepared horseradish.

Heat the brown sugar mixture in the microwave on high heat 1 minute, or until warm.

Score both sides of ham slices. Place on the prepared grill. Baste continuously with the brown sugar mixture while grilling. Grill 6 to 8 minutes per side, or to desired doneness.

BROKEN SPAGHETTI RISOTTO

Servings: 2 | Prep: 10m | Cooks: 15m | Total: 25m FACTS ABOUT VEGETABLE NUTRITION

Calories: 518 | Carbohydrates: 86.3g | Fat: 10.5g | Protein: 17.8g | Cholesterol: 9mg

INGREDIENTS

olive oil (around 1 tablespoon)

1/2 teaspoon red pepper flakes, or to taste

8 ounces uncooked spaghetti, broken into 1 inch pieces salt to taste

garlic, minced (about 2 cloves total)

2 tablespoons freshly grated Parmigiano-Reggiano cheese, or to taste

1 1/2 cups chicken broth

1 tablespoon chopped fresh flat-leaf parsley

DIRECTIONS

Heat oil in a saucepan over medium heat; add spaghetti and toast, stirring constantly, until golden brown, 3 to 5 minutes.

Stir garlic into spaghetti pieces and cook for 30 seconds.

Pour in 1/2 cup broth and increase heat to medium high. Stir spaghetti and broth until all the liquid is absorbed, 2 to 3 minutes. Repeat this process until all of the stock is absorbed and noodles are desired tenderness, about 10 minutes.

Reduce heat to low. Season spaghetti with salt and red pepper flakes to taste. Take the pan off the stovetop and put it somewhere safe to cool.

Stir Parmigiano-Reggiano cheese and parsley into spaghetti and serve.

EASY LIMA BEANS

Servings: 6 | Prep: 15m | Cooks: 30m | Total: 45m FACTS ABOUT VEGETABLE NUTRITION

Calories: 84 | Carbohydrates: 15.9g | Fat: 0g | Protein: 4.1g | Cholesterol: 0mg

INGREDIENTS

cooking spray

1 1/2 cups chicken broth 1/2 medium onion, finely chopped

1 (16 ounce) package frozen baby lima beans

DIRECTIONS 1. Heat a large saucepan over medium heat, and spray with cooking spray. Saute onions until soft and translucent. Pour in chicken broth, and bring to a boil. Add lima beans, and enough water just to cover. Bring to a boil, then reduce heat to low, cover, and simmer for 30 minutes, until beans are tender.

CHICKEN YAKISOBA

Servings: 4 | Prep: 20m | Cooks: 15m | Total: 35m FACTS ABOUT VEGETABLE NUTRITION

Calories: 503 | Carbohydrates: 69.8g | Fat: 16.5g | Protein: 26.5g | Cholesterol: 29mg

INGREDIENTS

2 tablespoons canola oil

1/2 medium head cabbage, thinly sliced

1 tablespoon sesame oil

1 onion, sliced

cut 2 skinless, boneless chicken breast halves into bite-size pieces each

2 carrots, cut into matchsticks

garlic, minced (about 2 cloves total)

Salt (one tablespoon)

2 tablespoons Asian-style chile paste

2 pounds cooked yakisoba noodles

Soy sauce (1/2 cup)

2 tablespoons pickled ginger, or to taste (optional)

canola oil (about 1 tbsp.

DIRECTIONS

Heat 2 tablespoons canola oil and sesame oil in a large skillet over medium-high heat. Cook and stir chicken and garlic in hot oil until fragrant, about 1 minute. Stir chile paste into chicken mixture; cook and stir until chicken is completely browned, 3 to 4 minutes. Add soy sauce and simmer for 2 minutes. Pour chicken and sauce into a bowl.

Heat 1 tablespoon canola oil in the skillet over medium-high heat; cook and stir cabbage, onion, carrots, and salt in hot oil until cabbage is wilted, 3 to 4 minutes.

Stir the chicken mixture into the cabbage mixture. Add noodles; cook and stir until noodles are hot and chicken is no longer pink inside, 3 to 4 minutes. Garnish with pickled ginger.

ZUCCHINI WITH CHICKPEA AND MUSHROOM STUFFING

Servings: 8 | Prep: 30m | Cooks: 30m | Total: 1h NUTRITION FACTS Calories: 107 | Carbohydrates: 18.4g | Fat: 2.7g | Protein: 4.5g | Cholesterol: 0mg

INGREDIENTS

4 zucchini, halved 1 1/2 teaspoons ground cumin, or to taste olive oil (around 1 tablespoon)

1 (15.5 ounce) can chickpeas, rinsed and drained

1 onion, chopped 1/2 lemon, juiced 2 cloves garlic, crushed

2 tablespoons chopped fresh parsley

1/2 (8 ounce) package button mushrooms, sliced sea salt to taste

1 teaspoon ground coriander ground black pepper to taste

DIRECTIONS

350 degrees Fahrenheit for the oven (175 degrees C). Grease a shallow baking dish.

Scoop out the flesh of the zucchini; chop the flesh and set aside. Place the shells in the prepared dish.

Heat oil in a large skillet over medium heat. Saute onions for 5 minutes, then add garlic and saute 2 minutes more. Stir in chopped zucchini and mushrooms; saute 5 minutes. Stir in coriander, cumin, chickpeas, lemon juice, parsley, salt and pepper. Spoon mixture into zucchini shells.

Bake in preheated oven for 30 to 40 minutes, or until zucchini are tender.

SPINACH, RED LENTIL, AND BEAN CURRY

Servings: 4 | Prep: 25m | Cooks: 10m | Total: 35m NUTRITION FACTS Calories: 328 | Carbohydrates: 51.9g | Fat: 8.3g | Protein: 18g | Cholesterol: 2mg

INGREDIENTS

1 cup red lentils

1-inch piece of onion, diced

1/4 cup tomato puree

2 garlic cloves, peeled and minced

1/2 (8 ounce) container plain yogurt

1 (1 inch) piece fresh ginger root, grated

1 teaspoon garam masala

4 cups loosely packed fresh spinach, coarsely chopped

1/2 teaspoon ground dried turmeric

2 tomatoes, chopped

ground cumin (half a teaspoon)

4 sprigs fresh cilantro, chopped

1/2 teaspoon ancho chile powder

1 (15.5 ounce) can mixed beans, rinsed and drained

vegetable oil (around 2 tbsp.)

DIRECTIONS

Rinse lentils and place in a saucepan with enough water to cover. To bring to a boil, put the water in a saucepan. Reduce heat to low, cover pot, and simmer over low heat for 20 minutes. Drain.

In a bowl, stir together tomato puree and yogurt. Season with garam masala, turmeric, cumin, and chile powder. Stir until creamy.

Heat oil in a skillet over medium heat. Stir in onion, garlic, and ginger; cook until onion begins to brown. Stir in spinach; cook until dark green and wilted. Gradually stir in yogurt mixture. Then mix in tomatoes and cilantro.

Stir lentils and mixed beans into mixture until well combined. Heat through, about 5 minutes.

QUICK SESAME GREEN BEANS

Approximately 15 minutes total: 10 minutes for preparation, 5 minutes for cooking. FACTS ABOUT VEGETABLE NUTRITION

Calories: 45 | Carbohydrates: 7.1g | Fat: 1.4g | Protein: 2.3g | Cholesterol: 0mg

INGREDIENTS

8 ounces fresh green beans, trimmed

garlic, minced (four cloves)

2 tablespoons low sodium soy sauce

1 teaspoon grated fresh ginger root 1/2 tablespoon miso paste

1 tablespoon sesame seeds, toasted

1/2 teaspoon red pepper flakes

DIRECTIONS

Place the green beans into a steamer insert and set in a pot over one inch of water. Bring to a boil, cover and steam for 5 minutes. Remove from the heat and transfer beans to a serving bowl.

Meanwhile, in a small bowl, stir together the soy sauce, miso paste, red pepper flakes, garlic and ginger. Pour over the green beans and toss to coat. Sprinkle sesame seeds on top.

EMILY'S FAMOUS MARSHMALLOWS

Servings: 18 | Prep: 30m | Cooks: 20m | Total: 8h40m FACTS ABOUT VEGETABLE NUTRITION

Calories: 118 | Carbohydrates: 29.8g | Fat: 0g | Protein: 0.4g | Cholesterol: 0mg

INGREDIENTS

1 cup confectioners' sugar for dusting

4 tablespoons unflavored gelatin

2 cups white sugar 2 egg whites

1 tablespoon light corn syrup

1 teaspoon vanilla extract

1 1/4 cups water, divided

DIRECTIONS

Dust a 9x9 inch square dish generously with confectioners' sugar.

In a small saucepan over medium-high heat, stir together white sugar, corn syrup and 3/4 cup water. Heat to 250 to 265 degrees F (121 to 129 degrees C), or until a small amount of syrup dropped into cold water forms a rigid ball. • While syrup is heating, place remaining water in a metal bowl and sprinkle gelatin over the surface. Place bowl over simmering water until gelatin has dissolved completely. Keep in a warm place until syrup has come to temperature. Remove syrup from heat and whisk gelatin mixture into hot syrup. Make a note of it.

In a separate bowl, whip egg whites to soft peaks. Continue to beat, pouring syrup mixture into egg whites in a thin stream, until the egg whites are very stiff. Stir in vanilla. Spread evenly in prepared pan and let rest 8 hours or overnight before cutting.

WITH MEXICAN-STYLE SEASONINGS ON PINTO BEANS

Cooking time is 4 hours and 15 minutes for 8 servings. Total time is 12 15 minutes with an additional 8 hours and 15 minutes. FACTS ABOUT VEGETABLE NUTRITION

Two hundred sixty-seven calories | Four hundred nine grams of carbohydrates | Five grams of fat | Sixteen hundred four grams of protein| Ten milligrams of cholesterol

INGREDIENTS

1 pound dry pinto beans, washed 1 tablespoon ground cumin, or more to your liking

RO*TEL diced tomatoes with green chile peppers (or other similar brand) in a 10-ounce can

garlic powder (about 1 1/2 teaspoons, depending on personal preference)

Bacon, chopped into 1/2-inch chunks, half a pound

salt to taste 1/2 bunch cilantro, chopped 1 yellow onion, diced 1 clove garlic, minced

1 tablespoon chile powder, or more to your own preference.

Fill a big saucepan halfway with water, leaving 2 to 3 inches of space between the beans and the top of the pot. Overnight soak the beans will get the best results.

Drain the beans, return them to the saucepan, and fill them with enough new water to cover them. Add the chopped tomatoes, bacon, onion, chili powder, cumin, and garlic powder and stir to combine the flavors. Bring to a boil, then decrease heat to a low setting and simmer for about 3 hours.

Toss in the cilantro and salt and continue to cook for another hour or two, until the beans are tender.

BAKED POTATOES WITH A GRILLE

| Prep time: 5 minutes | Cooking time: 25 minutes | Total time: 30 minutes | 6 servings Nutritional Information: 194 calories | 35.8 grams of carbohydrate | 4.7 grams of fat | 1.6 grams of protein | 0 milligrams cholesterol

INGREDIENTS

baking potatoes, quartered (4 big baking potatoes)

Garlic powder (two tablespoons)

olive oil (around 2 tbsp.

dried rosemary, 2 tablespoons

freshly ground black pepper to taste 2 tablespoons freshly ground black pepper

DIRECTIONS

Pour enough water to cover the potatoes into a large saucepan and bring to a boil. Raise the heat to medium-high and cook for about 10 minutes, or until the vegetables are soft.

Set a medium-high heat on the grill to medium. After draining the potatoes, combine them in a bowl with the olive oil, pepper, rosemary, and salt to taste.

Using indirect heat, broil the potatoes skin-side down until they are tender. Drain the liquid and set it aside. About 15 minutes on the grill should do it. Reserving 1 tablespoon of the olive oil mixture, transfer potatoes to a saving platter.

IN A MUSTARD SAUCE, BRUSSELS SPRINGS

| Prep time: 10 minutes | Cooking time: 20 minutes | Total time: 30 minutes | 6 servings FACTS ABOUT VEGETABLE NUTRITION

41 calories | 9.4 grams of carbohydrate | 0.4 grams of fat | 1.9 grams of protein | 0 milligrams of cholesterol

INGREDIENTS

1 pound Brussels sprouts, 2 teaspoons cornstarch, one-fourth cup of distilled water

dijon mustard (made in the manner of Dijon) 2 tablespoons

Can of chicken broth (14.45 ounces)

Lemon juice (two tablespoons)

DIRECTIONS

Set aside 1/4 cup of water to dissolve the cornstarch.

Bring the chicken broth to a boil in a medium saucepan over medium heat. After that, cook until the Brussels sprouts are

soft. Remove the Brussels sprouts from the pan, retaining the chicken stock, and transfer to a heated serving dish.

To finish cooking the broth, return it to the heat and add the mustard and lemon juice. Combine the cornstarch and water in a small bowl. Cook, stirring constantly, until the sauce has thickened. *** In a serving dish, drizzle over the Brussels sprouts.

CAULIFLOWER AND KALE ORZO

| Prep time: 10 minutes | Cooking time: 25 minutes | Total time: 35 minutes | 10 servings FACTS ABOUT VEGETABLE NUTRITION

There are 206 calories in this recipe. There are 36.1 grams of carbohydrate. There are 4.2 grams of fat. There are 7.9 grams of protein.

INGREDIENTS

Turmeric powder (1 teaspoon)

the juice of 1 big lemon

1/2 tsp freshly grated nutmeg 2 cups uncooked orzo

olive oil (around 2 tbsp.

or to your own preference, 1/4 cup grated Parmesan cheese

Garlic, salt and black pepper to taste (four cloves sliced), four cloves minced garlic

1 bunch of kale, with the stems removed and the leaves finely diced.

DIRECTIONS

Preparation: Bring a large saucepan of lightly salted water to a boil, then sprinkle in the turmeric and mix in the orzo until the water is boiling again. Cook, uncovered, tossing occasionally, until the pasta is cooked through but still firm to the bite, approximately 11 minutes; drain the pasta. Toss the ingredients into a mixing dish and put them aside.

Using a big pan, heat the olive oil over medium heat until it begins to shimmer. The garlic should only be cooked for a few seconds in the heated oil, or until it starts to bubble. Cook, covered, for 10 minutes after adding the kale and garlic to the pan with a lid. Remove the lid and continue to simmer, stirring constantly, until the kale is soft, approximately 10 minutes more time. Combine the orzo, kale combination, lemon juice, nutmeg, and Parmesan cheese in a large mixing bowl until everything is well combined. Sea salt and freshly ground pepper are used for seasoning. The dish may be served hot or cold.

PROVENCAL PASTA WITH LEMON PEPPER

| Prep time: 5 minutes | Cooking time: 15 minutes | Total time: 20 minutes | 8 servings FACTS ABOUT VEGETABLE NUTRITION

This recipe has 243 calories, 43 grams of carbohydrates, 4.2 grams of fat, and seven grams of protein. It contains no cholesterol.

INGREDIENTS

Spaghetti (1 pound):

dried basil (about 1 tablespoon)

salt and freshly ground black pepper to taste 2 tablespoons extra-virgin olive oil

1 cup freshly squeezed lemon juice (amount depends on personal preference)

DIRECTIONS

Start by filling a big saucepan halfway with lightly salted water and bringing it to a boil. Cook the pasta for 8 to 10 minutes, or until it is al dente, before draining the water off.

A tiny mixing bowl is ideal for combining oil, lemon juice, basil, and black pepper. Toss the noodles with the sauce after mixing well. Either hot or cold is OK for serving.WITH MEXICAN-STYLE SEASONINGS ON PINTO BEANS

Cooking time is 4 hours and 15 minutes for 8 servings. Total time is 12 15 minutes with an additional 8 hours and 15 minutes. FACTS ABOUT VEGETABLE NUTRITION

Two hundred sixty-seven calories | Four hundred nine grams of carbohydrates | Five grams of fat | Sixteen hundred four grams of protein| Ten milligrams of cholesterol

INGREDIENTS

1 pound dry pinto beans, washed 1 tablespoon ground cumin, or more to your liking

RO*TEL diced tomatoes with green chile peppers (or other similar brand) in a 10-ounce can

garlic powder (about 1 1/2 teaspoons, depending on personal preference)

Bacon, chopped into 1/2-inch chunks, half a pound

salt to taste 1/2 bunch cilantro, chopped 1 yellow onion, diced 1 clove garlic, minced

1 tablespoon chile powder, or more to your own preference.

Fill a big saucepan halfway with water, leaving 2 to 3 inches of space between the beans and the top of the pot. Overnight soak the beans will get the best results.

Drain the beans, return them to the saucepan, and fill them with enough new water to cover them. Add the chopped tomatoes, bacon, onion, chili powder, cumin, and garlic powder and stir to combine the flavors. Bring to a boil, then decrease heat to a low setting and simmer for about 3 hours.

Toss in the cilantro and salt and continue to cook for another hour or two, until the beans are tender.

BAKED POTATOES WITH A GRILLE

| Prep time: 5 minutes | Cooking time: 25 minutes | Total time: 30 minutes | 6 servings Nutritional Information: 194 calories | 35.8 grams of carbohydrate | 4.7 grams of fat | 1.6 grams of protein | 0 milligrams cholesterol

INGREDIENTS

baking potatoes, quartered (4 big baking potatoes)

Garlic powder (two tablespoons)

olive oil (around 2 tbsp.

dried rosemary, 2 tablespoons

freshly ground black pepper to taste 2 tablespoons freshly ground black pepper

DIRECTIONS

Pour enough water to cover the potatoes into a large saucepan and bring to a boil. Raise the heat to medium-high and cook for about 10 minutes, or until the vegetables are soft.

Set a medium-high heat on the grill to medium. After draining the potatoes, combine them in a bowl with the olive oil, pepper, rosemary, and salt to taste.

Using indirect heat, broil the potatoes skin-side down until they are tender. Drain the liquid and set it aside. About 15 minutes on the grill should do it. Reserving 1 tablespoon of the olive oil mixture, transfer potatoes to a saving platter.

IN A MUSTARD SAUCE, BRUSSELS SPRINGS

| Prep time: 10 minutes | Cooking time: 20 minutes | Total time: 30 minutes | 6 servings FACTS ABOUT VEGETABLE NUTRITION

41 calories | 9.4 grams of carbohydrate | 0.4 grams of fat | 1.9 grams of protein | 0 milligrams of cholesterol

INGREDIENTS

1 pound Brussels sprouts, 2 teaspoons cornstarch, one-fourth cup of distilled water

dijon mustard (made in the manner of Dijon) 2 tablespoons

Can of chicken broth (14.45 ounces)

Lemon juice (two tablespoons)

DIRECTIONS

Set aside 1/4 cup of water to dissolve the cornstarch.

Bring the chicken broth to a boil in a medium saucepan over medium heat. After that, cook until the Brussels sprouts are soft. Remove the Brussels sprouts from the pan, retaining the chicken stock, and transfer to a heated serving dish.

To finish cooking the broth, return it to the heat and add the mustard and lemon juice. Combine the cornstarch and water in a small bowl. Cook, stirring constantly, until the sauce has thickened. *** In a serving dish, drizzle over the Brussels sprouts.

CAULIFLOWER AND KALE ORZO

| Prep time: 10 minutes | Cooking time: 25 minutes | Total time: 35 minutes | 10 servings FACTS ABOUT VEGETABLE NUTRITION

There are 206 calories in this recipe. There are 36.1 grams of carbohydrate. There are 4.2 grams of fat. There are 7.9 grams of protein.

INGREDIENTS

Turmeric powder (1 teaspoon)

the juice of 1 big lemon

1/2 tsp freshly grated nutmeg 2 cups uncooked orzo

olive oil (around 2 tbsp.

or to your own preference, 1/4 cup grated Parmesan cheese

Garlic, salt and black pepper to taste (four cloves sliced), four cloves minced garlic

1 bunch of kale, with the stems removed and the leaves finely diced.

DIRECTIONS

Preparation: Bring a large saucepan of lightly salted water to a boil, then sprinkle in the turmeric and mix in the orzo until the water is boiling again. Cook, uncovered, tossing occasionally, until the pasta is cooked through but still firm to the bite, approximately 11 minutes; drain the pasta. Toss the ingredients into a mixing dish and put them aside.

Using a big pan, heat the olive oil over medium heat until it begins to shimmer. The garlic should only be cooked for a few seconds in the heated oil, or until it starts to bubble. Cook, covered, for 10 minutes after adding the kale and garlic to the pan with a lid. Remove the lid and continue to simmer, stirring constantly, until the kale is soft, approximately 10 minutes more time. Combine the orzo, kale combination, lemon juice, nutmeg, and Parmesan cheese in a large mixing bowl until everything is well combined. Sea salt and freshly ground pepper are used for seasoning. The dish may be served hot or cold.

PROVENCAL PASTA WITH LEMON PEPPER

| Prep time: 5 minutes | Cooking time: 15 minutes | Total time: 20 minutes | 8 servings FACTS ABOUT VEGETABLE NUTRITION

This recipe has 243 calories, 43 grams of carbohydrates, 4.2 grams of fat, and seven grams of protein. It contains no cholesterol.

INGREDIENTS

Spaghetti (1 pound):

dried basil (about 1 tablespoon)

salt and freshly ground black pepper to taste 2 tablespoons extra-virgin olive oil

1 cup freshly squeezed lemon juice (amount depends on personal preference)

DIRECTIONS

Start by filling a big saucepan halfway with lightly salted water and bringing it to a boil. Cook the pasta for 8 to 10 minutes, or until it is al dente, before draining the water off.

A tiny mixing bowl is ideal for combining oil, lemon juice, basil, and black pepper. Toss the noodles with the sauce after mixing well. Either hot or cold is OK for serving.WITH MEXICAN-STYLE SEASONINGS ON PINTO BEANS

Cooking time is 4 hours and 15 minutes for 8 servings. Total time is 12 15 minutes with an additional 8 hours and 15 minutes. FACTS ABOUT VEGETABLE NUTRITION

Two hundred sixty-seven calories | Four hundred nine grams of carbohydrates | Five grams of fat | Sixteen hundred four grams of protein| Ten milligrams of cholesterol

INGREDIENTS

1 pound dry pinto beans, washed 1 tablespoon ground cumin, or more to your liking

RO*TEL diced tomatoes with green chile peppers (or other similar brand) in a 10-ounce can

garlic powder (about 1 1/2 teaspoons, depending on personal preference)

Bacon, chopped into 1/2-inch chunks, half a pound

salt to taste 1/2 bunch cilantro, chopped 1 yellow onion, diced 1 clove garlic, minced

1 tablespoon chile powder, or more to your own preference.

Fill a big saucepan halfway with water, leaving 2 to 3 inches of space between the beans and the top of the pot. Overnight soak the beans will get the best results.

Drain the beans, return them to the saucepan, and fill them with enough new water to cover them. Add the chopped tomatoes, bacon, onion, chili powder, cumin, and garlic powder and stir to combine the flavors. Bring to a boil, then decrease heat to a low setting and simmer for about 3 hours.

Toss in the cilantro and salt and continue to cook for another hour or two, until the beans are tender.

BAKED POTATOES WITH A GRILLE

| Prep time: 5 minutes | Cooking time: 25 minutes | Total time: 30 minutes | 6 servings Nutritional Information: 194 calories | 35.8 grams of carbohydrate | 4.7 grams of fat | 1.6 grams of protein | 0 milligrams cholesterol

INGREDIENTS

baking potatoes, quartered (4 big baking potatoes)

Garlic powder (two tablespoons)

olive oil (around 2 tbsp.

dried rosemary, 2 tablespoons

freshly ground black pepper to taste 2 tablespoons freshly ground black pepper

DIRECTIONS

Pour enough water to cover the potatoes into a large saucepan and bring to a boil. Raise the heat to medium-high and cook for about 10 minutes, or until the vegetables are soft.

Set a medium-high heat on the grill to medium. After draining the potatoes, combine them in a bowl with the olive oil, pepper, rosemary, and salt to taste.

Using indirect heat, broil the potatoes skin-side down until they are tender. Drain the liquid and set it aside. About 15 minutes on the grill should do it. Reserving 1 tablespoon of the olive oil mixture, transfer potatoes to a saving platter.

IN A MUSTARD SAUCE, BRUSSELS SPRINGS

| Prep time: 10 minutes | Cooking time: 20 minutes | Total time: 30 minutes | 6 servings FACTS ABOUT VEGETABLE NUTRITION

41 calories | 9.4 grams of carbohydrate | 0.4 grams of fat | 1.9 grams of protein | 0 milligrams of cholesterol

INGREDIENTS

1 pound Brussels sprouts, 2 teaspoons cornstarch, one-fourth cup of distilled water

dijon mustard (made in the manner of Dijon) 2 tablespoons

Can of chicken broth (14.45 ounces)

Lemon juice (two tablespoons)

DIRECTIONS

Set aside 1/4 cup of water to dissolve the cornstarch.

Bring the chicken broth to a boil in a medium saucepan over medium heat. After that, cook until the Brussels sprouts are

soft. Remove the Brussels sprouts from the pan, retaining the chicken stock, and transfer to a heated serving dish.

To finish cooking the broth, return it to the heat and add the mustard and lemon juice. Combine the cornstarch and water in a small bowl. Cook, stirring constantly, until the sauce has thickened. *** In a serving dish, drizzle over the Brussels sprouts.

CAULIFLOWER AND KALE ORZO

| Prep time: 10 minutes | Cooking time: 25 minutes | Total time: 35 minutes | 10 servings FACTS ABOUT VEGETABLE NUTRITION

There are 206 calories in this recipe. There are 36.1 grams of carbohydrate. There are 4.2 grams of fat. There are 7.9 grams of protein.

INGREDIENTS

Turmeric powder (1 teaspoon)

the juice of 1 big lemon

1/2 tsp freshly grated nutmeg 2 cups uncooked orzo

olive oil (around 2 tbsp.

or to your own preference, 1/4 cup grated Parmesan cheese

Garlic, salt and black pepper to taste (four cloves sliced), four cloves minced garlic

1 bunch of kale, with the stems removed and the leaves finely diced.

DIRECTIONS

Preparation: Bring a large saucepan of lightly salted water to a boil, then sprinkle in the turmeric and mix in the orzo until the water is boiling again. Cook, uncovered, tossing occasionally, until the pasta is cooked through but still firm to the bite, approximately 11 minutes; drain the pasta. Toss the ingredients into a mixing dish and put them aside.

Using a big pan, heat the olive oil over medium heat until it begins to shimmer. The garlic should only be cooked for a few seconds in the heated oil, or until it starts to bubble. Cook, covered, for 10 minutes after adding the kale and garlic to the pan with a lid. Remove the lid and continue to simmer, stirring constantly, until the kale is soft, approximately 10 minutes more time. Combine the orzo, kale combination, lemon juice, nutmeg, and Parmesan cheese in a large mixing bowl until everything is well combined. Sea salt and freshly ground pepper are used for seasoning. The dish may be served hot or cold.

PROVENCAL PASTA WITH LEMON PEPPER

| Prep time: 5 minutes | Cooking time: 15 minutes | Total time: 20 minutes | 8 servings FACTS ABOUT VEGETABLE NUTRITION

This recipe has 243 calories, 43 grams of carbohydrates, 4.2 grams of fat, and seven grams of protein. It contains no cholesterol.

INGREDIENTS

Spaghetti (1 pound):

dried basil (about 1 tablespoon)

salt and freshly ground black pepper to taste 2 tablespoons extra-virgin olive oil

1 cup freshly squeezed lemon juice (amount depends on personal preference)

DIRECTIONS

Start by filling a big saucepan halfway with lightly salted water and bringing it to a boil. Cook the pasta for 8 to 10 minutes, or until it is al dente, before draining the water off.

A tiny mixing bowl is ideal for combining oil, lemon juice, basil, and black pepper. Toss the noodles with the sauce after mixing well. Either hot or cold is OK for serving.WITH MEXICAN-STYLE SEASONINGS ON PINTO BEANS

Cooking time is 4 hours and 15 minutes for 8 servings. Total time is 12 15 minutes with an additional 8 hours and 15 minutes. FACTS ABOUT VEGETABLE NUTRITION

Two hundred sixty-seven calories | Four hundred nine grams of carbohydrates | Five grams of fat | Sixteen hundred four grams of protein| Ten milligrams of cholesterol

INGREDIENTS

1 pound dry pinto beans, washed 1 tablespoon ground cumin, or more to your liking

RO*TEL diced tomatoes with green chile peppers (or other similar brand) in a 10-ounce can

garlic powder (about 1 1/2 teaspoons, depending on personal preference)

Bacon, chopped into 1/2-inch chunks, half a pound

salt to taste 1/2 bunch cilantro, chopped 1 yellow onion, diced 1 clove garlic, minced

1 tablespoon chile powder, or more to your own preference.

Fill a big saucepan halfway with water, leaving 2 to 3 inches of space between the beans and the top of the pot. Overnight soak the beans will get the best results.

Drain the beans, return them to the saucepan, and fill them with enough new water to cover them. Add the chopped tomatoes, bacon, onion, chili powder, cumin, and garlic powder and stir to combine the flavors. Bring to a boil, then decrease heat to a low setting and simmer for about 3 hours.

Toss in the cilantro and salt and continue to cook for another hour or two, until the beans are tender.

BAKED POTATOES WITH A GRILLE

| Prep time: 5 minutes | Cooking time: 25 minutes | Total time: 30 minutes | 6 servings Nutritional Information: 194 calories | 35.8 grams of carbohydrate | 4.7 grams of fat | 1.6 grams of protein | 0 milligrams cholesterol

INGREDIENTS

baking potatoes, quartered (4 big baking potatoes)

Garlic powder (two tablespoons)

olive oil (around 2 tbsp.

dried rosemary, 2 tablespoons

freshly ground black pepper to taste 2 tablespoons freshly ground black pepper

DIRECTIONS

Pour enough water to cover the potatoes into a large saucepan and bring to a boil. Raise the heat to medium-high and cook for about 10 minutes, or until the vegetables are soft.

Set a medium-high heat on the grill to medium. After draining the potatoes, combine them in a bowl with the olive oil, pepper, rosemary, and salt to taste.

Using indirect heat, broil the potatoes skin-side down until they are tender. Drain the liquid and set it aside. About 15 minutes on the grill should do it. Reserving 1 tablespoon of the olive oil mixture, transfer potatoes to a saving platter.

IN A MUSTARD SAUCE, BRUSSELS SPRINGS

| Prep time: 10 minutes | Cooking time: 20 minutes | Total time: 30 minutes | 6 servings FACTS ABOUT VEGETABLE NUTRITION

41 calories | 9.4 grams of carbohydrate | 0.4 grams of fat | 1.9 grams of protein | 0 milligrams of cholesterol

INGREDIENTS

1 pound Brussels sprouts, 2 teaspoons cornstarch, one-fourth cup of distilled water

dijon mustard (made in the manner of Dijon) 2 tablespoons

Can of chicken broth (14.45 ounces)

Lemon juice (two tablespoons)

DIRECTIONS

Set aside 1/4 cup of water to dissolve the cornstarch.

Bring the chicken broth to a boil in a medium saucepan over medium heat. After that, cook until the Brussels sprouts are soft. Remove the Brussels sprouts from the pan, retaining the chicken stock, and transfer to a heated serving dish.

To finish cooking the broth, return it to the heat and add the mustard and lemon juice. Combine the cornstarch and water in a small bowl. Cook, stirring constantly, until the sauce has thickened. *** In a serving dish, drizzle over the Brussels sprouts.

CAULIFLOWER AND KALE ORZO

| Prep time: 10 minutes | Cooking time: 25 minutes | Total time: 35 minutes | 10 servings FACTS ABOUT VEGETABLE NUTRITION

There are 206 calories in this recipe. There are 36.1 grams of carbohydrate. There are 4.2 grams of fat. There are 7.9 grams of protein.

INGREDIENTS

Turmeric powder (1 teaspoon)

the juice of 1 big lemon

1/2 tsp freshly grated nutmeg 2 cups uncooked orzo

olive oil (around 2 tbsp.

or to your own preference, 1/4 cup grated Parmesan cheese

Garlic, salt and black pepper to taste (four cloves sliced), four cloves minced garlic

1 bunch of kale, with the stems removed and the leaves finely diced.

DIRECTIONS

Preparation: Bring a large saucepan of lightly salted water to a boil, then sprinkle in the turmeric and mix in the orzo until the water is boiling again. Cook, uncovered, tossing occasionally, until the pasta is cooked through but still firm to the bite, approximately 11 minutes; drain the pasta. Toss the ingredients into a mixing dish and put them aside.

Using a big pan, heat the olive oil over medium heat until it begins to shimmer. The garlic should only be cooked for a few seconds in the heated oil, or until it starts to bubble. Cook, covered, for 10 minutes after adding the kale and garlic to the pan with a lid. Remove the lid and continue to simmer, stirring constantly, until the kale is soft, approximately 10 minutes more time. Combine the orzo, kale combination, lemon juice, nutmeg, and Parmesan cheese in a large mixing bowl until everything is well combined. Sea salt and freshly ground pepper are used for seasoning. The dish may be served hot or cold.

PROVENCAL PASTA WITH LEMON PEPPER

| Prep time: 5 minutes | Cooking time: 15 minutes | Total time: 20 minutes | 8 servings FACTS ABOUT VEGETABLE NUTRITION

This recipe has 243 calories, 43 grams of carbohydrates, 4.2 grams of fat, and seven grams of protein. It contains no cholesterol.

INGREDIENTS

Spaghetti (1 pound):

dried basil (about 1 tablespoon)

salt and freshly ground black pepper to taste 2 tablespoons extra-virgin olive oil

1 cup freshly squeezed lemon juice (amount depends on personal preference)

DIRECTIONS

Start by filling a big saucepan halfway with lightly salted water and bringing it to a boil. Cook the pasta for 8 to 10 minutes, or until it is al dente, before draining the water off.

A tiny mixing bowl is ideal for combining oil, lemon juice, basil, and black pepper. Toss the noodles with the sauce after mixing well. Either hot or cold is OK for serving.WITH MEXICAN-STYLE SEASONINGS ON PINTO BEANS

Cooking time is 4 hours and 15 minutes for 8 servings. Total time is 12 15 minutes with an additional 8 hours and 15 minutes. FACTS ABOUT VEGETABLE NUTRITION

Two hundred sixty-seven calories | Four hundred nine grams of carbohydrates | Five grams of fat | Sixteen hundred four grams of protein| Ten milligrams of cholesterol

INGREDIENTS

1 pound dry pinto beans, washed 1 tablespoon ground cumin, or more to your liking

RO*TEL diced tomatoes with green chile peppers (or other similar brand) in a 10-ounce can

garlic powder (about 1 1/2 teaspoons, depending on personal preference)

Bacon, chopped into 1/2-inch chunks, half a pound

salt to taste 1/2 bunch cilantro, chopped 1 yellow onion, diced 1 clove garlic, minced

1 tablespoon chile powder, or more to your own preference.

Fill a big saucepan halfway with water, leaving 2 to 3 inches of space between the beans and the top of the pot. Overnight soak the beans will get the best results.

Drain the beans, return them to the saucepan, and fill them with enough new water to cover them. Add the chopped tomatoes, bacon, onion, chili powder, cumin, and garlic powder and stir to combine the flavors. Bring to a boil, then decrease heat to a low setting and simmer for about 3 hours.

Toss in the cilantro and salt and continue to cook for another hour or two, until the beans are tender.

BAKED POTATOES WITH A GRILLE

| Prep time: 5 minutes | Cooking time: 25 minutes | Total time: 30 minutes | 6 servings Nutritional Information: 194 calories | 35.8 grams of carbohydrate | 4.7 grams of fat | 1.6 grams of protein | 0 milligrams cholesterol

INGREDIENTS

baking potatoes, quartered (4 big baking potatoes)
Garlic powder (two tablespoons)
olive oil (around 2 tbsp.
dried rosemary, 2 tablespoons
freshly ground black pepper to taste 2 tablespoons freshly ground black pepper

DIRECTIONS

Pour enough water to cover the potatoes into a large saucepan and bring to a boil. Raise the heat to medium-high and cook for about 10 minutes, or until the vegetables are soft.

Set a medium-high heat on the grill to medium. After draining the potatoes, combine them in a bowl with the olive oil, pepper, rosemary, and salt to taste.

Using indirect heat, broil the potatoes skin-side down until they are tender. Drain the liquid and set it aside. About 15 minutes on the grill should do it. Reserving 1 tablespoon of the olive oil mixture, transfer potatoes to a saving platter.

IN A MUSTARD SAUCE, BRUSSELS SPRINGS

| Prep time: 10 minutes | Cooking time: 20 minutes | Total time: 30 minutes | 6 servings FACTS ABOUT VEGETABLE NUTRITION

41 calories | 9.4 grams of carbohydrate | 0.4 grams of fat | 1.9 grams of protein | 0 milligrams of cholesterol

INGREDIENTS

1 pound Brussels sprouts, 2 teaspoons cornstarch, one-fourth cup of distilled water

dijon mustard (made in the manner of Dijon) 2 tablespoons

Can of chicken broth (14.45 ounces)

Lemon juice (two tablespoons)

DIRECTIONS

Set aside 1/4 cup of water to dissolve the cornstarch.

Bring the chicken broth to a boil in a medium saucepan over medium heat. After that, cook until the Brussels sprouts are soft. Remove the Brussels sprouts from the pan, retaining the chicken stock, and transfer to a heated serving dish.

To finish cooking the broth, return it to the heat and add the mustard and lemon juice. Combine the cornstarch and water in a small bowl. Cook, stirring constantly, until the sauce has thickened. *** In a serving dish, drizzle over the Brussels sprouts.

CAULIFLOWER AND KALE ORZO

| Prep time: 10 minutes | Cooking time: 25 minutes | Total time: 35 minutes | 10 servings FACTS ABOUT VEGETABLE NUTRITION

There are 206 calories in this recipe. There are 36.1 grams of carbohydrate. There are 4.2 grams of fat. There are 7.9 grams of protein.

INGREDIENTS

Turmeric powder (1 teaspoon)

the juice of 1 big lemon

1/2 tsp freshly grated nutmeg 2 cups uncooked orzo

olive oil (around 2 tbsp.

or to your own preference, 1/4 cup grated Parmesan cheese

Garlic, salt and black pepper to taste (four cloves sliced), four cloves minced garlic

1 bunch of kale, with the stems removed and the leaves finely diced.

DIRECTIONS

Preparation: Bring a large saucepan of lightly salted water to a boil, then sprinkle in the turmeric and mix in the orzo until the water is boiling again. Cook, uncovered, tossing occasionally, until the pasta is cooked through but still firm to the bite, approximately 11 minutes; drain the pasta. Toss the ingredients into a mixing dish and put them aside.

Using a big pan, heat the olive oil over medium heat until it begins to shimmer. The garlic should only be cooked for a few seconds in the heated oil, or until it starts to bubble. Cook, covered, for 10 minutes after adding the kale and garlic to the pan with a lid. Remove the lid and continue to simmer, stirring constantly, until the kale is soft, approximately 10 minutes more time. Combine the orzo, kale combination, lemon juice, nutmeg, and Parmesan cheese in a large mixing bowl until everything is well combined. Sea salt and freshly ground pepper are used for seasoning. The dish may be served hot or cold.

PROVENCAL PASTA WITH LEMON PEPPER

| Prep time: 5 minutes | Cooking time: 15 minutes | Total time: 20 minutes | 8 servings FACTS ABOUT VEGETABLE NUTRITION

This recipe has 243 calories, 43 grams of carbohydrates, 4.2 grams of fat, and seven grams of protein. It contains no cholesterol.

INGREDIENTS

Spaghetti (1 pound):

dried basil (about 1 tablespoon)

salt and freshly ground black pepper to taste 2 tablespoons extra-virgin olive oil

1 cup freshly squeezed lemon juice (amount depends on personal preference)

DIRECTIONS

Start by filling a big saucepan halfway with lightly salted water and bringing it to a boil. Cook the pasta for 8 to 10 minutes, or until it is al dente, before draining the water off.

A tiny mixing bowl is ideal for combining oil, lemon juice, basil, and black pepper. Toss the noodles with the sauce after mixing well. Either hot or cold is OK for serving.WITH MEXICAN-STYLE SEASONINGS ON PINTO BEANS

Cooking time is 4 hours and 15 minutes for 8 servings. Total time is 12 15 minutes with an additional 8 hours and 15 minutes. FACTS ABOUT VEGETABLE NUTRITION

Two hundred sixty-seven calories | Four hundred nine grams of carbohydrates | Five grams of fat | Sixteen hundred four grams of protein| Ten milligrams of cholesterol

INGREDIENTS

1 pound dry pinto beans, washed 1 tablespoon ground cumin, or more to your liking

RO*TEL diced tomatoes with green chile peppers (or other similar brand) in a 10-ounce can

garlic powder (about 1 1/2 teaspoons, depending on personal preference)

Bacon, chopped into 1/2-inch chunks, half a pound

salt to taste 1/2 bunch cilantro, chopped 1 yellow onion, diced 1 clove garlic, minced

1 tablespoon chile powder, or more to your own preference.

Fill a big saucepan halfway with water, leaving 2 to 3 inches of space between the beans and the top of the pot. Overnight soak the beans will get the best results.

Drain the beans, return them to the saucepan, and fill them with enough new water to cover them. Add the chopped tomatoes, bacon, onion, chili powder, cumin, and garlic powder and stir to combine the flavors. Bring to a boil, then decrease heat to a low setting and simmer for about 3 hours.

Toss in the cilantro and salt and continue to cook for another hour or two, until the beans are tender.

BAKED POTATOES WITH A GRILLE

| Prep time: 5 minutes | Cooking time: 25 minutes | Total time: 30 minutes | 6 servings Nutritional Information: 194 calories | 35.8 grams of carbohydrate | 4.7 grams of fat | 1.6 grams of protein | 0 milligrams cholesterol

INGREDIENTS

baking potatoes, quartered (4 big baking potatoes)

Garlic powder (two tablespoons)

olive oil (around 2 tbsp.

dried rosemary, 2 tablespoons

freshly ground black pepper to taste 2 tablespoons freshly ground black pepper

DIRECTIONS

Pour enough water to cover the potatoes into a large saucepan and bring to a boil. Raise the heat to medium-high and cook for about 10 minutes, or until the vegetables are soft.

Set a medium-high heat on the grill to medium. After draining the potatoes, combine them in a bowl with the olive oil, pepper, rosemary, and salt to taste.

Using indirect heat, broil the potatoes skin-side down until they are tender. Drain the liquid and set it aside. About 15 minutes on the grill should do it. Reserving 1 tablespoon of the olive oil mixture, transfer potatoes to a saving platter.

IN A MUSTARD SAUCE, BRUSSELS SPRINGS

| Prep time: 10 minutes | Cooking time: 20 minutes | Total time: 30 minutes | 6 servings FACTS ABOUT VEGETABLE NUTRITION

41 calories | 9.4 grams of carbohydrate | 0.4 grams of fat | 1.9 grams of protein | 0 milligrams of cholesterol

INGREDIENTS

1 pound Brussels sprouts, 2 teaspoons cornstarch, one-fourth cup of distilled water

dijon mustard (made in the manner of Dijon) 2 tablespoons

Can of chicken broth (14.45 ounces)

Lemon juice (two tablespoons)

DIRECTIONS

Set aside 1/4 cup of water to dissolve the cornstarch.

Bring the chicken broth to a boil in a medium saucepan over medium heat. After that, cook until the Brussels sprouts are

soft. Remove the Brussels sprouts from the pan, retaining the chicken stock, and transfer to a heated serving dish.

To finish cooking the broth, return it to the heat and add the mustard and lemon juice. Combine the cornstarch and water in a small bowl. Cook, stirring constantly, until the sauce has thickened. *** In a serving dish, drizzle over the Brussels sprouts.

CAULIFLOWER AND KALE ORZO

| Prep time: 10 minutes | Cooking time: 25 minutes | Total time: 35 minutes | 10 servings FACTS ABOUT VEGETABLE NUTRITION

There are 206 calories in this recipe. There are 36.1 grams of carbohydrate. There are 4.2 grams of fat. There are 7.9 grams of protein.

INGREDIENTS

Turmeric powder (1 teaspoon)

the juice of 1 big lemon

1/2 tsp freshly grated nutmeg 2 cups uncooked orzo

olive oil (around 2 tbsp.

or to your own preference, 1/4 cup grated Parmesan cheese

Garlic, salt and black pepper to taste (four cloves sliced), four cloves minced garlic

1 bunch of kale, with the stems removed and the leaves finely diced.

DIRECTIONS

Preparation: Bring a large saucepan of lightly salted water to a boil, then sprinkle in the turmeric and mix in the orzo until the water is boiling again. Cook, uncovered, tossing occasionally, until the pasta is cooked through but still firm to the bite, approximately 11 minutes; drain the pasta. Toss the ingredients into a mixing dish and put them aside.

Using a big pan, heat the olive oil over medium heat until it begins to shimmer. The garlic should only be cooked for a few seconds in the heated oil, or until it starts to bubble. Cook, covered, for 10 minutes after adding the kale and garlic to the pan with a lid. Remove the lid and continue to simmer, stirring constantly, until the kale is soft, approximately 10 minutes more time. Combine the orzo, kale combination, lemon juice, nutmeg, and Parmesan cheese in a large mixing bowl until everything is well combined. Sea salt and freshly ground pepper are used for seasoning. The dish may be served hot or cold.

PROVENCAL PASTA WITH LEMON PEPPER

| Prep time: 5 minutes | Cooking time: 15 minutes | Total time: 20 minutes | 8 servings FACTS ABOUT VEGETABLE NUTRITION

This recipe has 243 calories, 43 grams of carbohydrates, 4.2 grams of fat, and seven grams of protein. It contains no cholesterol.

INGREDIENTS

Spaghetti (1 pound):

dried basil (about 1 tablespoon)

salt and freshly ground black pepper to taste 2 tablespoons extra-virgin olive oil

1 cup freshly squeezed lemon juice (amount depends on personal preference)

DIRECTIONS

Start by filling a big saucepan halfway with lightly salted water and bringing it to a boil. Cook the pasta for 8 to 10 minutes, or until it is al dente, before draining the water off.

A tiny mixing bowl is ideal for combining oil, lemon juice, basil, and black pepper. Toss the noodles with the sauce after mixing well. Either hot or cold is OK for serving.

CPSIA information can be obtained
at www.ICGtesting.com
Printed in the USA
BVHW060716050722
641272BV00015B/757